# CANCER RECOVERY

# CANCER RECOVERY

## A Daily Program to
## Heal Cancer Naturally

### Ayurveda,
### Metabolic Enzymes
### &
### The New Medicine

Raven Jones

*Certified Ayurvedic Practitioner & Cancer Survivor*

Cancer Recovery Press
P.O.Box 1752
Sebastopol, CA 95473

Printed in the United States of America

ISBN: 978-0-578-06310-2

*Dedicated to*

*Elizabeth 'Bobsy' Draper*

*1941 – 2001*

# Disclaimer

This book details the author's personal experiences with and opinions about cancer. Although the author, Raven Jones, has attempted to give a profound understanding of the topics discussed and to ensure accuracy and completeness of any information that originates from any other source than his own, he and the publisher assume no responsibility for errors, inaccuracies, omissions, or any inconsistency herein. This book is not intended to replace the advice and treatment of a physician who specializes in the treatment of diseases. It is essential that before you begin any healthcare program, or change your lifestyle in any way, you consult your physician, oncologist or other licensed healthcare provider to ensure that you are in good health and that examples contained in this book will not harm you. The statements and claims made about products and services have not been evaluated by the U.S. Food and Drug Administration. They are not intended to treat, diagnose, cure, or prevent any condition or disease.

This book provides content related to topics concerning physical and/or mental health issues. As such, use of this book implies your acceptance of this disclaimer.

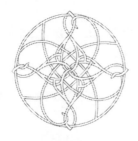

# CONTENTS

# PART III: THE PROGRAM

# PART IV: THE SOUL

# PART V: THE SENSES

# ACKNOWLEDGEMENTS

I would like to thank the following people who have contributed to my health and the writing of this book: Akara Draper, for her trust and support when I needed it. Frank Lobsiger, for his wisdom and guidance. Walter Orion, for his playfulness and strength. Orchid and Gabriel for making me a proud father. Chase Davis for our walks and talks. Karen Parrish for teaching me about persistence, Janice Manov for her generosity of Spirit. Ambika Copple, Della Davis and all my fellow students at the Mount Madonna College of Ayurveda. Dr. Vasant Lad, for his foundational teachings. Ashtavaidyan Alathiyoor Narayanan Nambi, Dr. Moos, Dr. Bosco, Dr. Devi Narayanan, Rupaaj and all the staff at the SNA Ayurveda Nursing Home in Thrissur, Kerala, India. Helene Gentili for her faith and Curandera wisdom. Dr. Salvador Vargas and the staff at Betania West, Tijuana, Mexico. Dr Issac Eliaz of the Amitabha Clinic for his commitment to healing his patients and me. Barton Stone, Constance Miles and Barbara Stavola for giving me love and community. Mina Balakhani for nursing me. Michele Newmark for making me breathe. Aubrey Degnan for her Presence and DeAnna Batdorff for her Inspiration. MaryShiela and Shanti for their eagle eye editing and finally Hillary Lynne for the cover design and fabulous illustrations.

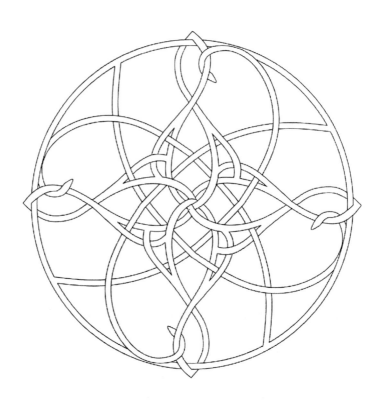

# COMMITMENT

Unless one is committed, there is hesitancy,
the chance to draw back, always ineffectiveness.
Concerning all acts of initiative (and creation),
there is one elemental truth, the ignorance of which
kills countless ideas and splendid plans.
That the moment one definitely commits oneself,
then providence moves, too.
All sorts of things occur to help one
that would never otherwise have occurred.
A whole stream of events issue forth from the discussion,
raising in one's favour all manner of unforeseen incidents
and meetings and material assistance, which no man
or woman could have dreamt
would have come their way.

W .H .Murray,
The Scottish Himalayan Expedition

# INTRODUCTION

## The Journey Through Cancer

I F you have been diagnosed with cancer, or if you are caring for someone who has cancer, and you are searching for some complimentary, natural, alternative healing options, then this book was written for you.

The information you will find in these pages may help you prevent or recover from any illness and is an invaluable guide for anyone seeking knowledge about health and wellness.

Maybe you have chosen the path of western allopathic medicine and want to supplement it with an integrative path combining natural, holistic methods. You may be scared about your prognosis and just beginning to come to terms with taking charge of your healing process. Or you may have reached the limits of what chemotherapy, radiation and surgery have to offer and you are looking for a miracle. In any case; do not despair; there is a way for you to begin to heal yourself *naturally*. You must only be open to discover it.

I myself was searching for a book like this when I was diagnosed with a malignant cancer tumor the size of a golf ball on my right knee. I was told that they needed to amputate my leg as soon as possible to prevent any further spread of the cancer. I was in shock, confused and angry. How could this happen to me? A fit outdoorsman in his late 50's who had led a very healthy life? I wasn't ready to die or even loose a limb. There had to be some mistake. I had made other plans. I want another flight please!

However, little did I know at the time, my life was about to change forever. Thus began my own search for healing and, after many difficult and amazing lessons, I decided to write this book to help others like me who are suddenly thrust into a health crisis and are searching for more natural ways to affect a cure.

There is an old saying that goes something like this...... "Sometimes the worst thing that can happen to you turns out to be the best thing that can happen; if you don't let it get the best of you." I am a cancer survivor now after my wife died of cancer nine years ago. I wish I had known then, when she became ill, what I know now; that there are many safe alternatives to western medicine if you know where to look. You just have to find the right ones for you.

Here I have chronicled my own journey through cancer, discovering alternative and complementary healing methods, diets and lifestyles that worked for me and others, so that you can make some informed choices for yourself. Along the way you will make your own discoveries and begin to take charge of your own healing process which is different from everyone else's. You must first decide if healing is really what you want more than anything else, because making that positive choice, whole-heartedly, is the beginning of your journey to health.

## ANYTHING CAN BE HEALED!

*"It is the Vital Life-Force that heals,*
*because dead men need no medicine."*
—Samuel Hahneman, Creator of Homeopathy

First let me say that I do not heal or cure cancer. Nobody heals cancer, but you can be *an active participant* in your body's efforts to heal itself. The only thing that can heal cancer is the *Vital Life Force* that is in you and pervades the universe and infuses all things. If by chance you choose a path of healing, whether it is Western Allopathic or Natural Alternative or a combination of both, that results in a healing, it is always the miraculous power of the body and God's Grace.

As the old saying goes, "God helps those who help themselves" and it is *your* participation in *your* healing and the cooperation of the miracle that is your physical body that often makes the difference between life and death.

So, dear One, choose Life and begin from this moment on to listen to your body and engage every vital cell in the process of achieving health. Others have healed from cancer with little or no participation in their own bodily process than absolute reliance on God. You can do more than this and increase your chances of becoming well again. Start today to open yourself up to however you personally connect to God or the Divine Conscious Awareness of Being and be open to see what transpires.

Whatever happens, be safe in the knowledge that you cannot fail, you can only complete your destiny and God willing, that will be new life and wellness. Remember that true health is not an event, it is a process. It took a long time and a certain set of circumstances for you to become so imbalanced that a physical symptom showed up to warn you of the danger if right action is not taken. Consequently, it will take some time and effort to correct the imbalance and return you to your natural state of true health.

This book is based on what I term the four pillars of the Natural Cancer Recovery Program :

1) *An Ayurvedic Lifestyle* which includes diet and nutritional supplementation.
2) *Detoxification* – cleansing the body of old toxins.
3) *Metabolic Enzymes* – A daily program of specific supplements.

**4)** <u>*The New Medicine*</u> – Healing the emotional conflicts underlying all diseases.

May the healing crisis that you are perhaps facing now, help you to appreciate the wonderful gift of Life. May you come to understand that the incredible miracle that is your body, knows how to heal itself and, with your help and the information in this book, you will begin the journey to wellness today.

Kerala, India

October, 2010

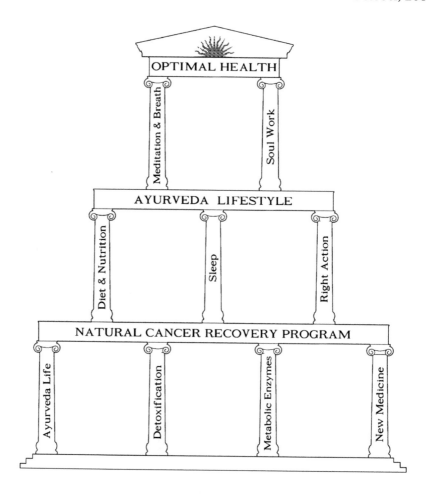

Figure 1: The Three Tiers of Ayurvedic Health

# FOREWORD

## LETTER FROM INDIA
## OCTOBER 6TH 2010

## NO PICNIC

Dearest friends

This morning I awoke in the half light to the sound of heavy rain, its incessant roar like the ocean waves as it pelted the giant coconut palms and banana leaves all around the Ayurveda clinic of this little village in Kerala, South West India. Outside comes the exotic wailing of the 'whoopo' birds and a barking dog complaining bitterly of his situation in the neighbor's yard not fifteen feet from my ground floor window, open wide to receive the cool breeze of the South East Monsoon.

It never rains but it pours would be the right expression to describe the intensity of the weather here, so extreme that all the buildings are stained with the moldy vegetation that grows happily in the steamy heat rising after the rains subside. This is my 4th annual visit to the small, traditional Ayurveda clinic and I am comfortably familiar with the sounds and smells of this ancient country. I have fallen in love with these handsome, coffee-skinned people, their jet black hair and smiling eyes, who waggle their heads in friendly greeting, animated and curious in their desire to know you.

The rain still cascades off the roof into large puddles along the walls outside and I think of Sita, the woman who is in charge of cleaning the rooms here. At this moment she is preparing to leave home in the dark. Everyday she rises at 4 am to make her family's breakfast and packed lunches before leaving the house for the 40 minute bus ride and half hour walk to arrive at the clinic by 8 am. At 5 pm she makes the reverse journey to prepare dinner and do her washing and cleaning before retiring to sleep at 10 pm until the cycle starts again. Like half of the population on this planet she makes only a few dollars a day.

I have been here 3 days now and my sleep cycle is just beginning to adjust to the 13 hour time difference. I had forgotten how intense the Ayurvedic treatments are and twice a day I reel back into my room to absorb the effects of the oil and herbs as my body responds to the medicine. Healing doesn't quite describe the feeling. Powerful, passionate, penetrating and deeply transforming on a cellular level is what it is. Sort of like the monsoon rain, now slackening off a little, as the water floods into the muddy gullies along the edges of the road.

It is 6.30 am and Anish arrives, with a knock at my door, to prepare my morning medicine, one of six I will take at various intervals throughout the day. Not a pleasant drink, something like old coffee gone wrong, but I welcome the chance to cleanse my body with its acrid taste. Anyway, breakfast will arrive soon with the large, thin, rice pancakes called **dosas** and the sweet, spicy coconut meal to dip them in.

Each time I come here I am healthier and it feels like any trace of cancer has been purged from my body by the relentless healing power of the Earth's natural plants. I have been restored and rejuvenated by the herbs and hands of Ayurveda India. It's no picnic here........... more like a grand feast of life and I want to share it with you!

# PART I

## THE MIND

### MY STORY AND
### WHAT I DISCOVERED
### ABOUT HEALING CANCER

*"All healing, all health comes from
the story you continually tell yourself."*
*Dr Christiane Northrup*
*'Women's Bodies Women's Wisdom'*

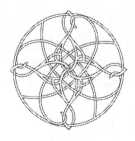

# CHAPTER 1

# WITH A LITTLE HELP
# FROM MY FRIENDS

*"The person who is not their own physician by the time they are forty, is a fool."*
Paracelsus,
Early 16th Century

"**H**EY! How are you doing Jonzoid?"

The familiar voice on the other end of the telephone called me by a nickname he had given me nearly 30 years ago. I hadn't seen Peter for a number of years and when I had called him a few months ago I was told he was in India studying Ayurveda. This is the traditional healing art of that country developed over 5,000 years ago, incorporating a way of living in balance with nature and providing a holistic system of healing using plant based medicine, diet, lifestyle, spiritual and emotional awareness that is still practiced widely in India and is now rapidly being discovered in America.

I told Peter about my cancer diagnosis and that I was recovering from an operation to remove a golf ball sized malignant tumor from my right knee.

"Well let me ask you a few questions" he said "what are you eating?"

I told him that I had been on a strict vegan diet for 6 months, mostly raw, incorporating vegetable juices and blended smoothies and that I was low in energy and had lost a lot of weight that I really couldn't afford to lose. It was winter, I lived Santa Cruz, California, close to the ocean in a damp little cottage and I had a hard time keeping warm but I felt I needed to purify my body to bring it back to health.

Peters' response was emphatic, "Stud!" he said, "You're eating the wrong food. You're like eating ice cream in Alaska. I know you, you're Vata, (an Ayurvedic body type, usually thin with a lot of nervous energy) you need to eat hot, soupy foods. Do you know what Kitcheree is?"

Actually, I did. It is an Indian dish made with basmati rice and split mung beans flavored with turmeric, cumin and mustard seeds. I told Peter that a local vegetarian restaurant served it everyday but I had not tried it.

"Well you need to go get some. Better still learn to make it yourself and start eating it everyday!"

This was only part of Peters' advice that day, but it was the beginning of a long journey that put me on the road to health and led to the writing of this book. I did learn to make Kitcheree and still eat it several times a week. As I learned more about the healing foods of Ayurveda I became fascinated by it's healing principles but it wasn't until a year and a half later that some other friends nudged me further in that direction.

I was sitting in my living room having a conversation with my two closest friends Walter and Frank. It was after the cancer had returned and I had traveled to Mexico for another operation to remove the new tumor. I was contemplating paying $2500 for a PET scan to see if there was any cancer still in my body. My Insurance Company had long since cancelled my policy and I would have to use my own hard earned money so I was doubly reluctant to pay to look for a cancer I didn't want to find.

My friends sat opposite me and they could see that I was anxious and irritable and unsure what to do. "What do you guys think?" I asked them.

"Well I have an idea," replied Frank. "What if you took the $2,500 you were going to spend on the PET scan and used it to travel to India for Pancha Karma cleansing. That way you would be pro-active in your healing process and the money would be well spent."

"You'd have a great adventure and discover more about Ayurveda, which you are interested in," chimed in Walter, who had himself been to India and knew something of its culture.

In that instant my whole mood changed as I saw the wisdom of Frank's idea. Ayurveda was fast becoming a part of my daily lifestyle. Here I had a chance to put its healing tools to the test in the birthplace of this ancient healing art. My whole being brightened up and a big smile creased my face, "What a great idea," I said. "I'm going to do it!"

Some months later I was on the long journey half way around the world to the Motherland of India to truly begin my healing experience. Shortly after I returned I became a student at the Mt Madonna College of Ayurveda in Watsonville, California, and eventually I became an Ayurvedic Practitioner.

What I discovered through this process and the subsequent 5 years of research into the many natural cancer cures, is that healing cancer is a very individual process. Just as no two human beings are the same, no two cancer cases are the same. One thing is true however, and that is each person must undertake a radical shift in their lifestyle. This means introducing a different diet which often includes more live foods and fewer or no animal products in the beginning, a specific nutritional supplement program and a course of detoxification and cleansing. The mind/body connection is addressed and the emotional component that is at the heart of all true healing.

After all this, nothing is guaranteed. It is up to the individual Soul to complete the journey to wellness on its own, by listening to what the body already knows............how to heal itself.

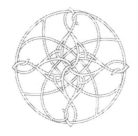

# CHAPTER 2

# WHOA! STOP EVERYTHING!

*"Nature makes the cure; the doctor's job is to aid nature"*
Hippocrates (400 BC)

"THIS is a very aggressive type of cancer and the best cure is to amputate your leg above the knee." The oncologist/surgeon looked at me sympathetically. I could see that he had done many amputations and this was just another day at work for him. I flashed on him using a big hacksaw to saw off my leg and I felt sick to my stomach.

I had come to this big hospital in San Francisco because an orthopedic surgeon in my home town of Santa Cruz had made what this oncologist described as an "oops!", a misdiagnosis basically, and according to him an all too common occurrence. The small town orthopedic surgeon had removed a large cyst on my right knee which had grown to the size of a golf ball without checking for cancer. "I've done hundreds of these. I can fit you in next Tuesday" is what he had boasted. But he had told me in a previous examination that because of the rapid growth, there was an outside chance that it could be a sarcoma cancer. Right there he should have referred me to a cancer oncologist or, at the very least, ordered a biopsy before proceeding.

The surgery went ahead and, ten days later, there was a call from the doctor's office. I had better come in. They had found something. The after surgery pathology report confirmed a very rare, aggressive form of sarcoma cancer. I was given several oncologists in San Francisco to call. Not only that, as the swelling from the operation went down, it revealed that a second tumor, caused by the mishandled surgery, had spread to the other side of my knee. Oops! indeed!

Here is the first lesson I learned. **_Always_** get a second opinion and a third, if necessary. Each doctor has different knowledge and experience. Find someone you would trust with your life. It's that important. Second lesson, **_always_** go to a major hospital in a big city and ask to see the best and most experienced oncologist they have. Get referrals if you can, and other patients' opinions about that doctor.

At this stage you are going to be given very little choice in the course of treatment. It will be either surgery, radiation or chemotherapy or all three; the big three, and the only three that conventional oncologists can offer you. And they are usually in a hurry! Listen to what they have to say. Don't panic. You will have a more stressful experience if you do. You have time. Go home and think about it. I mean _really_ meditate on it. You have been given an opportunity here and the decisions you make now may affect the rest of your life. Do some research into the alternatives, get help with this...... B-r-e-a-t-h-e.

In my ignorance I didn't do this. Now I know better. I had found this experienced oncologist and he had to perform two more operations to repair the damage of the "oops!" However, he wasn't totally successful and because of the damage previously done he uttered those dreaded words "We weren't able to get it all". Meaning, that because the tumor was so close to the bone the margins of safety were not achieved and there were still cancer cells left in the tissue of the muscle.

To make matters worse, Blue Cross, my insurance company, was retroactively canceling my recent policy because of a technicality to do with my eyes. Apparently it is standard procedure to investigate claims on new policies to catch any pre-existing conditions. There weren't any, but they had found a loophole in a small box I had not checked about my eyes - anything apparently, to get out of paying for my expensive surgery.

I chose to try a 7 week course of radiation, with the risk that the tumor could return. I told the doctor about my lack of funds for the treatment, and he blithely told me that amputation was cheaper than radiation, if I wanted to change my mind. I could not believe he had said that and told him so. As I left the hospital that day I looked at the other patients lined up behind me. Some were on crutches with only one leg. Many were in wheelchairs. All the people in the waiting area looked sick and tired and afraid. When I went out of the big revolving doors and stood in the street outside, I made a vow to myself. "I'm never going back in there! I am going to find another way."

It took five long years of research, trial and error on my journey to wellness. I have tried many alternative healing methods. At one stage I was taking 12 different natural medicines each morning. This book is a catalogue of most of what I tried and then some more that I have heard from other survivors. I hope this book will give you the information and inspiration that I so desperately needed when I came out of that hospital.

Whether you decide to use only natural alternatives or an integrated, complementary approach, as I did at first, use the information and resources that I have compiled here to explore your own path. What worked for me won't necessarily work for you. We are all uniquely individual in our mental, spiritual and physiological design. But we do have one thing in common, a desire to be well. May the following chapters inform and inspire you. May you begin the first steps on your path to wellness by taking charge of your own healing.

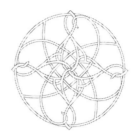

# CHAPTER 3

# TIME OUT

*"The loss of illusion may be the beginning of wisdom."*

Dr. Ralph Moss

**Questioning Chemotherapy**

IF the first lesson of healing is to always get a second opinion, and the second lesson is to choose a major hospital for surgery, the third lesson is the title of the previous chapter, "Whoa! Stop Everything!" The reason that a symptom of disease has appeared somewhere in the body in the form of cancer is a message screaming to be heard. The deeper message is usually that something about the way that you are living has thrown the body/mind out of balance. It is never too late to address that imbalance. So now, what can be done?

Often the diagnosis comes as a severe shock to the system. Fear, doubt and confusion crowd out any coherent thoughts. Very often this first stage of the healing crisis is accompanied by hospital tests and waiting for results. This can be a harrowing time. Make sure you have family or trusted friends accompany you to the doctor's meetings. They can be your advocates and because it is not their diagnosis or test results, they will be able to take notes and ask questions that you may not think of. They will be able to integrate the reality of the situation that fear often prevents you from doing. Taking notes helps sort out the diagnostic medical information and keeps track of your options.

Beware, at this early stage, of a rush to action. Doctors should have your best interests at heart but are conditioned to act quickly and may want to rush you into surgery within days according to their busy schedules. At this very important moment, take some time to think it over. Sleep on it for a few days. This is when to take a *'time out'*, to stop everything, get quiet and survey your options. A week or two will give you time to make realistic choices.

In my own case a teacher of mine told me I should go home and sit on the couch for a week and do nothing. "Just stare at the walls," he said, "and wait for information to come to you." It was good advice. I stopped answering the phone and checking my email. I stopped listening to the daily news. It allowed me to face my own fears and get a little objective distance, so I could begin to hear what my body was saying and weigh the alternative choices.

This time out does not sit well with most oncologists. Their first reaction is one of frustration. They can be patronizing and discourage you from taking the power of decision away from them. They believe that they know what's best for you. They may tell you how important it is to act without delay, but no matter how seriously advanced the disease is, a few days or a week will not make such a difference and it could help to change the course of your healing process in a positive way before it is too late to have a choice. There is no wrong action here, even if you choose to follow the doctors' advice. However, a time out gives you a chance for a second opinion even if it is only your own.

This is when to start your research and seek out people, like me and other Cancer Researchers, who have information to share. Call on friends to research the internet for you and have your main advocate read the books and articles, filter the information and forward you interesting options. This can be an overwhelming time, with so many people concerned and wanting to help. Ultimately there are several inexpensive actions you can take to begin your healing process right away. You will feel immediately empowered!

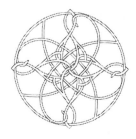

# CHAPTER 4

# THE LAW OF FLOW

*To those who are good to me. I am good.*
*To those who are not good to me.*
*I am also good.*
*Thus, all experience good.*
*To those who are sincere with me.*
*I am sincere.*
*To those who are not sincere with me.*
*I am also sincere.*
*Thus, all experience sincerity.*

Lao Tsu

YOU'VE been diagnosed with cancer, now what? In China when people are diagnosed with cancer they are sent to bed for a month of bed rest with herbal treatments while a course of action is determined. Here in the United States patients with manageable symptoms are usually told to continue their life as normal while routine tests and minor procedures are performed. This may be an economic hardship for most people with jobs and family to support, but, this is the very time to stop and review your lifestyle. What has caused the disease to appear in your body? Your system is out of its healthy, immunological balance which we all take for granted every day. So what has changed and what is your body trying to tell you?

If at all possible take time off work. Stop the busyness. Retreat to a quiet place for reflection, which may mean just staying at home and resting. Take some contemplative walks in nature, if you are feeling well enough. If not, take some medication for pain to give you some breathing space and just sit. Sit on the couch in a quiet room where you won't be disturbed and let the mind run until it quiets down. Try not to worry. This is a very productive time no matter how it looks. Information will come. This is not unlike meditation, but if you're not familiar with this practice, allow yourself to just rest. Take naps, talk with your loved ones, take stock of your life. As a teacher of mine says, "Just do the next obvious thing

During this time, and particularly if you are undergoing the first few months of treatment or rehabilitation, find time to be alone. Turn off the T.V. and cancel the newspapers. Don't subject yourself to any negative input whether from TV news reports, violent movies, or other media sensationalism. The world will get along just fine without you monitoring it. This kind of input is exactly the kind of stress you want to eliminate from your life. On the other hand, do by all means, create harmony and joy in your life. Listen to music that is healing and harmonious. Read inspirational books and novels.

Stay away from computers and cell phones. Let someone else take the calls and report the news. You don't want to have to confirm your diagnosis and treatment over and over to well meaning friends and relatives. Check out for a while, your friends will understand. Leave an upbeat, grateful message on your answering machine. Speak to people you want to only when you have the time and energy to do so without taxing yourself.

This time is for you and everyone around you has to know this.

Be clear with friends and family about your needs and wants. They will be glad to comply, just as you would if the situation was reversed. If you want to research your health issues, delegate it to someone else. There will be plenty of offers to help. Start learning to receive the support and care you need.

Taking time out will give you insight and intuitive messages which you then can act on. Only from here can you make informed and conscious choices about the method of treatment you want to pursue, whatever that may be.

Remember, if you want to get well, *things will have to change drastically.* Stop thinking you can muddle along with your regular life and handle your disease on the side. Your life is not going to be normal for a while. Get committed to change for the better. The sooner you do this, the sooner you will feel confident about your own healing process. When the mind becomes positive, the body will respond likewise. Giving yourself this time out from your usual life is just the beginning of the positive changes that will keep you healthy for the rest of your life.

Here I want to add a caveat. Whatever brings you joy in your life, continue to do that. If that is non-stressful work that you love or the family you care for as a mother or father, keep being useful and positive, without over taxing yourself. The immune system thrives on an upbeat and engaged life of creativity. This can also be a way to promote your healing response. By the same token, if you have a tendency to depression and fear, then the immune system will struggle to fight any disease that may be waging war in your body. Do what it takes to bring aliveness into your life at the same time honoring the body's need to rest and heal.

Sleep is sometimes the best medicine. The Japanese have a saying, *"Two hours sleep before midnight is worth four after"*, meaning, get to bed early even if it isn't your tendency and if you are experiencing insomnia try Melatonin, a naturally occurring hormone that helps to promote sleep. This is especially good if you are undergoing radiation or chemotherapy treatments. Or, if you are milk tolerant, take a glass of warm milk before bed and add a pinch each of cardamom, nutmeg and cinnamon (freshly ground if possible) , add a little honey to taste.

The body wants to get well but you must cooperate with it. If you are tired during the day don't fight it. Allow time for naps. Tiredness will come and go in cycles. Just know that your energy will return in due course.

# Trust the Law of Flow

Have you ever been late for an appointment and you are driving a little too fast? Whenever I experience this, it always teaches me the same lesson. No matter how I try to get there faster by overtaking or trying to beat traffic lights, I always get delayed. All the lights are red or I get behind the slowest driver in the universe. A giant truck is backing out into the road ahead or it pulls out in front of me. It seems the faster I try to go, the more obstacles are thrown in my way.

The reverse is also true. If I am early for an appointment with plenty of time to spare, everything opens up for me. All the traffic lights turn green as I drive effortlessly through them. The road is clear and the more relaxed I am, the easier my drive. I usually slow down more and get there with 10 minutes to spare. I call this the Law of Flow.

You can apply this law to your cancer diagnosis. Everything seems speeded up and overwhelming. There are 'red lights' everywhere and big decisions blocking your way. You may feel that you are going to be late for your healing if you don't get things done quickly. But there is information you need out there, just waiting for you to slow down and receive it. I encourage you to slow down, and take the time to listen to your intuition and 'give the road ahead time to clear'. Let go and know that there are lessons here for you to receive, so that the healing process can begin. Wait for the lights to turn green as you approach your health choices. Trust the Law of Flow.

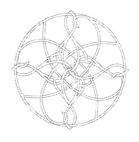

CHAPTER 5

# SOMEDAY

*"Tell me, what is it you plan to do, with your one wild and precious life?"*
Mary Oliver

MOST cancer patients who have survived talk about a significant shift that occurred in their life because of the illness. Life will never be quite the same again and that's a good thing. When illness strikes, your whole routine goes out the window and, besides being profoundly disrupting, your sickness is a sign that something you were doing, or the way you were living, was out of balance.

It may not have been obvious before but when we become ill our bodies are trying to tell us something. Now it has got to this drastic stage because we weren't listening. Perhaps we noticed signs or symptoms early on but didn't take heed. Could we have suppressed an alarm signal that was demanding change? What was it in your lifestyle that was out of balance? Maybe stress in your lifestyle, job or relationships was taking its toll on your physical and mental heath? Perhaps like me you have suffered a great loss in your life.

Maybe diet and environmental chemicals have accumulated too many toxins in your body? Was your life going nowhere? Were you depressed or over anxious about money, family or work? Sometimes, illness can strike like a bolt out of the blue into a normal, healthy, young life and there is no rhyme or reason to it. In any case it is not, at this stage, useful to regret or wish things had been different. What is needed is a complete lifestyle change!

"Wait!" you say, "I don't have to change anything. My life was perfect." Well how perfect could it have been if you've ended up sick? Now is the time for revision and revolution. Most long term cancer survivors, no matter what course of healing they chose, decided early on that they were going to get well no matter what it took. Attitude is paramount. Even if you feel beaten down and sideswiped by this turn of events in your life, positivity is the key. These survivors also made big changes in their lives. Something wasn't working even if, at least on the surface, everything seemed great. There is a deeper lesson to be learned here. So don't miss this opportunity. If you make no changes and decide to continue on as before, there is a chance that another lesson may come along that is harder than the first one.

Start to ask the hard questions. Keep a journal and record feelings that arise. Here is what a client of mine did to record her journey with breast cancer. I have changed her name for privacy reasons and reprint something she wrote with her permission. Nancy started a 'blog' with CaringBridge.org, an online website for people with illness to keep in touch with their friends. This way she was able to express her feelings in her own time. This is a passage from her blog.

*" I am full of questions these days: How do we know what matters to us? How does one know what would make them glad to get up in the morning, and what it is that would be an absorbing event that allows one to go to bed "good" and tired? How does one know what they love—especially when one has spent years not listening to the protests of one's body, ignored one's feelings, over-ridden one's dreams, or gone about ignoring other messages of deep unhappiness?*
*Such questions on a beautiful, sunny day in California... what I am realizing in this moment is, a life threatening illness that brings life to a full stop can be soul serving, if it involves the inner practice of asking and finding daily answers to these questions. So today, I ask myself, am I*

*going to do something that I <u>want</u> to do? Am I going to spend a moment doing something that I <u>love</u> to do, today? Am I going to follow my instincts, allowing what I love to show its face to me? Will I <u>nourish</u> my soul today?"*

This is a profoundly inspiring passage for anyone to read. This is what true healing is about. Take stock, slow down, and listen deeply. What do you want most in your life? What has been missing that you have sacrificed for something else? It may be to start doing all those things that you have dreamed you would do 'someday', Someday when I retire. Someday, when I have enough money. Someday, when the kids are finished college. Someday, when I find the love of my life. We don't have a lot of time! We are only here for an instant in the great span of infinity. You *will* die. If not this time, then eventually, because as the song by Jackson Brown goes, "All good things, gotta come to an end."

The moment you begin to take responsibility for your own healing and live with the conviction that you will change for the better, the healing process will start to work on some level. Start making a difference in your relationships now. Be discriminating and cut out those people in your life who make you feel worse. Be compassionate with these people, but take charge of your new life, and get to work to make amends with the things that will lead you to perfect health again.

Simplify your life. Give stuff away. We all have a basement or a closet full of things we don't need. Renew friendships on a deeper level. Tell people you love them, *every day!* Be honest with yourself. What will you do to make a difference if you are given the chance to be well again? The **attitude of gratitude** is the single, most powerful road to happiness and healing that I know. I saw a bumper sticker once that said "Don't Postpone Joy." Too often we are waiting for things to happen *to* us. Begin today to take charge of your healing process.

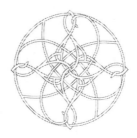

# CHAPTER 6

# CREATING A SUPPORT TEAM

**O**NE of the most helpful things to support positive healing energy during an illness, is to build a team of family and friends to take care of all your needs. This is particularly true after a major operation. If we have family living with us, they'll be worrying about your diagnosis and the projected outcome. They need support too. Before a scheduled operation it is good to enlist the help of a close friend, one you know is capable and a good organizer. It is important that they are willing to help. Some friends and even family members will not be able to be there for you. Don't take it personally. Many people fear illness and death, and cancer has its own stigma.

Some friends will not call or may be to be too busy with their own lives to be available to you. Sometimes because of their own natural fear of hospitals and surgery they will make excuses why they cannot help or visit. This is a time when true friends stay connected. You may discover friends you didn't even know you had. There will be one or two who have the time and inclination to be your 'Team Leader'. This person should <u>not</u> be your spouse no matter how willing they may be. Spouses/partners are stressed enough caring for you. They also will need the support you are going to ask for.

One of the most beneficial things that your team leader can do for you is to organize meals. Their job will be to call a list of people that you think may be willing to help. Don't be shy. Giving people the opportunity to serve is a gift in itself. Ask them to prepare and deliver a lunch or a dinner once a week for the next three or four weeks. Ask them to make their favorite dishes, based on the diet you want to eat. Not only does this feed you and your family, it also affords a time for visiting and sharing food, if and when you want company. This will be for you to decide, depending upon your appetite and energy level. You may just want them to drop it off when convenient, then it can be refrigerated for later use.

I have found that most friends, when contacted personally by the team leader, are grateful for the chance to serve and can usually bring food at least once when requested, even if it is purchased from a favorite restaurant or deli.

The bigger the list of helpers the better, but a team of 6 or 7 people can supply at least one hot meal a day. They may even ask if there is more that they can do. Accept this offer gracefully and keep an emergency list for times when help is needed: running errands, additional housework, laundry, home cooking, child care etc. This kind of help can be invaluable in the first few weeks of recovery. It can also include rides to the doctor's office or the hospital for treatments.

If you feel any tendency toward negativity or hysteria from friends, it is important to take a break from their company. Clear all negativity and fearful emotions from your environment. This doesn't mean that things have to be superficially hyper-positive and unrealistic. Sometimes the best way for people to be with you is to just sit in silence and hold your hand or read a book. Just spending quiet time together can be the most helpful support for your healing journey.

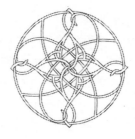

CHAPTER 7

# SUPPORT FOR
# THE CANCER PATIENT

*"Surround yourself with positive people and ideas."*

Raven Jones

SUPPORT groups are only helpful if they are supporting your way of healing. Unfortunately, most cancer support groups set up by major hospitals are for patients only on the traditional western medical path of chemotherapy, radiation and surgery. They will talk about their previous and upcoming operations and chemo treatments with knowledgeable technical language while munching on sugar cookies and donuts and sipping sodas and coffee. If you are interested in an alternative route, this is not in your best interests. It is best to avoid them. They may not understand your reasoning and may even excoriate you for wanting to try something different, because this approach contradicts their own choices.

It may not be easy to find people who are using an alternative, holistic approach to healing, or even an integrated one, combining western and alternative modalities. Search on line or place an ad in a local weekly to find others of like interest. Put an ad up on a local community bulletin board. Some therapists hold regular support groups for people facing serious health challenges. These would be more suitable to you.

I found many supportive people in the Mexican clinics that I visited, because some of the treatments that I wanted to try have been banned in the USA by the American Medical Association and the Food and Drug Administration. For nearly 40 years now it has been illegal for any M.D. in the USA to treat cancer with anything other than chemotherapy, radiation or surgery. They can loose their license. Indeed, history is full of the suppression of alternative medicine by the AMA, in league with the large pharmaceutical and insurance industries. Many good doctors and health practitioners who have used inexpensive cures have been harassed and threatened, sometimes by armed enforcement officers. Their practices and lives have been ruined and some have even been jailed or forced to take their practice across the border to Mexico.

From California I traveled to Tijuana, Mexico to find the clinic of Dr. Salvador Vargas. Almost all of his patients had gone there as a last resort after undergoing months and even years of surgeries and chemotherapy. Many of these patients, were being treated with low dose, cyto-static, target-specific chemotherapy and radiation. This is one fifth of the amount administered in the U.S. The chemotherapy is also combined with other healing modalities such as high doses of multi-vitamins in I.V. form along with liquid laetrile and amino acid combinations. Many were very supportive in the relaxed atmosphere of the I.V. room and I received many good tips on treatments and therapies that had helped other people. They told of their own discoveries of alternative medicine and the information, often referrals, that had led them to Dr. Vargas' clinic.

Steer clear of anyone who is fearful or negative about your choices. Only keep company with those who are supporting your decision, whatever that may be. Surround yourself with life-supporting people and ideas.

Over the six months of my treatment visits I met many families with amazing stories of both failure and success. Some of the patients were too far advanced to be helped, but all had an indomitable spirit to be well. Some of these brave people I would never see again, but there were also many success stories, including mine.

Many did recover and managed to reverse the negative side effects of the massive doses of toxic chemicals they had received. During visits to other clinics in Tijuana I heard many stories of people being poorly treated by western doctors and finally told that there was nothing more that could be done to help them. It was usually at this stage that they turned to alternatives and, sometimes, it was too late to reverse the damage that had already been done.

If at all possible start using complementary treatments along with your conventional medicine or commit to alternative holistic medicines right from the beginning. Whatever you decide - and there is no right or wrong - trust in what you are doing and allow the treatment to work on you. If, at some point, you want to stop or change treatments, listen to your deep, intuitive self. Your body knows what it needs to heal itself. You will intuit which action to take when you become still enough to hear the message.

Cancer has a huge stigma attached to it. People are not always sure how to talk about it. They often want to know what kind of cancer you have so that they can relate to it and put it in a box based on the information they have about it. People would often ask me with some fear and dread, "Is the cancer gone?". At first I would explain what the latest test results said but this was invariably negative. Then I began to say in a Pollyanna fashion, which I only superficially believed, " I am healthy and getting better every day in every way!" This didn't convince anyone, including me, and seemed to even disappoint some who fed on bad news. Eventually I realized that the best mind/body choice was to state truthfully: I really didn't know if the cancer had gone but I felt I was getting better, and I was grateful to be living day by day.

When I stopped getting tests to prove I had cancer, my mind was more relaxed and positive. Why would I go looking for something I didn't want to find? I didn't have to know what the doctors' prognosis was and therefore I was able to live more positively and follow my own healing path into a brighter future.

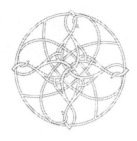

# CHAPTER 8

# CARING FOR THE CAREGIVER

*"I am aware of floating through time and space*
*gifted with the bounties of the journey*
*yet never owning any of them.*
*It is like living in a dream*
*where everything seems real, solid,*
*and yet we are, all of us -*
*leaves, toads, humans -*
*just passing through."*

Alice Walker

WHEN one suffers from debilitating illness, many people may mobilize to support you. Friends and family often step up and begin to take extra care of you. Your needs, naturally, become paramount. In this rush to help, the caregivers can become selfless in their desire to help you back to health. Herein lies a much unacknowledged fact. The primary caregiver, especially if it is a spouse or close member of your family, takes second place where needs are concerned. Often these unsung heroes are overlooked when all the attention is focused upon you, the sick person.

In fact, the caregiver often feels worse off than you - not only do they have to reorganize their lives to suit your needs, but they can feel helpless, scared, anxious and, very often, guilty too. They may feel terrible emotional pain, watching you suffer through the illness and treatments while they remain healthy. Sometimes the caregiver becomes the sole breadwinner too, and this compounds the stress.

It is important to recognize emotions that they may wish to hide from you the patient. It is best for them to let these feelings surface right from the beginning. Once fears and doubts are acknowledged between you and your loved ones, it makes it easier to confront the journey together and to construct a positive plan of action.

If you are a caregiver reading this, make sure you are getting your needs met too. Be straight forward if you are becoming overwhelmed and seek professional help from a counselor. Ask friends and family to sub for you from time to time and take a break. Go somewhere away from the duties at home. Get a massage or spend time with friends and talk about yourself. The more you are rested and taken care of yourself, the more available you will be for your loved one. Self-care for caregivers is of utmost importance.

# A LOVE STORY

I met Bobsy in Oakland, California, on a bright, sunny day in mid July. She was 56 years old and I was 54. She was a beautiful, intelligent, healthy outdoors woman from Boston, living in Santa Cruz, California. We were both attending the same Spiritual Retreat and I first saw her at a lunch break, as many of the attendees sat on the grass lawn outside enjoying the sun. She was sitting cross-legged, on the grass in a circle of women, talking animatedly. She had perfect posture and wore beautiful clothes and I knew right away that I wanted to be a friend of this intriguing woman. It took me a few days to drum up the courage to introduce myself, but we found out later it was love at first sight for both of us.

We had both been alone for many years, unable to find anyone who was right for us, so we had determined to live alone rather than settle for any thing less than our hearts' desire. After we got together, we were in a whirlwind of love, albeit tempered by our years of maturity which was telling us to go slow. We never quarreled and spent almost every hour together in blissful happiness. Before long we bought a fixer-upper and moved in, planning a long and fruitful life together.

On the 2nd anniversary of our first meeting we planned to get engaged to be married. A week before the event she discovered a lump the size of a pea in her breast. She was a cancer survivor, having healed from breast cancer in the other breast seven years before. At that time she had undergone traditional surgery, radiation and chemotherapy.

We put our best faces on and went ahead with the engagement party where Bobsy told everyone and asked for their prayers. We determined to fight this thing together. Bobsy underwent radiation again and several alternative treatments but nothing would stop the spread of the cancer in her lungs. Then she developed a second cancer in the form of a sarcoma tumor on her scapular followed by surgery, more radiation and a desperate last ditch visit to an alternative clinic in Florida. Only a short nine months after our engagement party, she was dead.

After a year of care giving and her subsequent death, I was exhausted and an emotional wreck. I took several months off work, but I was in a state of shock. I felt guilty about her going instead of me and, on some level I didn't want to live without her. The pain of her loss was too hard to bear. I suppressed my grief and tried to move on with my life. It was less than 2 years later that I was diagnosed with the same rare sarcoma that she had developed, and I entered my own healing crisis.

Many questions arose for me. Was my cancer caused by the trauma of Bobsy's death? Was my failure to feel the grief of her loss a cause for the breakdown of my immune system? Were there emotional factors in my inheritance of her property and my guilt about deserving it? Was it my lack of will to live without her or my anger about her being taken from me so soon? Why did I get the same one-in-one million, rare form of cancer that she had?

There have been studies done about the most common occurrences of cancer in people who had received traumatic events in their lives. These are the top five:

1) Death of a spouse or child

2) Loss of career or job

3) Divorce

4) Sudden loss of fortune

5) Sudden gain of fortune

It is clear to me in retrospect, that Bobsy's death threw me into such an emotional turmoil, that I was unable to process the grief, anger, and abandonment that I felt at her loss. It was only several years later, while dealing with my own cancer, that I began to realize the consequences of not being able to release my own emotional turmoil around her loss.

As a preventative measure, and particularly when healing from cancer, always seek counseling around the traumatic events in your life. Learn to deeply feel the emotions that arise and how to process them. They say a therapist is an expensive friend, so talk with friends about it, too. Keep a journal of your daily thoughts and feelings. If you are a caregiver, seek regular help to process unexpressed emotions. Putting a brave face on things may seem to help the person you are supporting but it doesn't help you. Find an outlet for grief, frustration or anger. It may save your life!

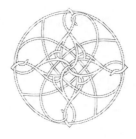

CHAPTER 9

# SURRENDER

*This is the day which God hath made.*
*Let us rejoice and be glad in it.*

Psalm 118

WHEN the diagnosis of cancer comes there is the initial shock, denial and often the rage and anger associated with any unwanted, personal intrusion into our way of life. What seems like an unwarranted attack on the physical body is often met with the determination to fight back. Family members and friends will assuage their fears by pledging their support in the ensuing battle and often with the accompanying cry of "We're going to beat this!"

Sometimes this all or nothing attitude helps the cancer patient put a positive spin on the future outlook. Armed with the heavy artillery of surgery, chemotherapy and radiation, they can meet the adversary head on and wage war. This falls in line with current western thinking on how to 'fight' cancer with such popular sayings as 'The Fight for The Cure' (or 'The War on Drugs' and 'The War on Terrorism') and, the all too familiar obituary.....,"After a long *battle* with cancer etc....." The idea of us against 'It' helps galvanize peoples attitudes toward funding the big cancer research institutions like the National Cancer Institute and The American Cancer Society in the 40 year search for a cure. But has this attitude helped us find a way to heal ourselves?

The woeful survival success rate (between 3 and 7% after five years), and skewed results of the large pharmaceutical corporations would suggest not. Here I want to recommend another way of looking at disease, and cancer in particular. All symptoms are the body's cry for attention. What we do next is important. Throwing oneself into the fight does give many people a sense of hope about a positive path to healing. Despite this rallying of the troops, in many cases they are fighting a losing battle. The immune system suffers irreparable damage from the attacks of chemotherapy and radiation, designed to poison and burn the cancer cells in the body.

What I am suggesting here is to look at cancer not as the enemy, but as a messenger. Not a messenger of doom, but a wake up call. Will we listen to the alarms being sounded by the symptoms that have changed the body's normal functioning? Do we want to kill this messenger and bomb it to oblivion before we have understood its message? I would ask you to consider being open to surrender to the circumstances that are unfolding before your eyes.

This does not mean passively waving a white flag and giving up. It means accepting the situation with as much calm and curiosity as possible. What is the body telling you? What does it need from you? How do you treat the cancer messenger? Perhaps it is actually the body's way of trying to protect itself and survive? In this case maybe "shooting first and asking questions later" is not the best method of healing.

This does not mean one should roll over and do nothing, although curiously enough, studies have shown this leads many people to live longer than those who seek aggressive treatment. In fact the martial art of Aikido can teach us something here about how to deal with a supposedly aggressive opponent. Rather than charging the symptoms head on, by stepping aside or re-directing the energy, we can take action to support the body's natural defenses and ask, what has caused this radical change in our health?

It is my belief that the 'cancer' stigma in modern society is so associated with fear and the fight against it, that we have forgotten to ask the question 'What caused this?' and more importantly 'How do I remove the cause?' From an Ayurvedic perspective the cause is almost always a question of the poor digestion and assimilation of the nutrients that feed and grow our bodies. Along with other pollutants that have entered our system from environmental poisons, to emotional and lifestyle stress, the eliminative organs have become overwhelmed and seriously depleted. So much so, that the resultant toxins have leaked into areas of the body where they shouldn't be. This toxic build up has resulted in the body's need to produce tumors and rapidly reproducing cells trying to contain the damage. *The 'bio-terrain' has become compromised.*

Therefore we must not obliterate this valuable information by putting more toxins in the body such as chemotherapy. We must take positive action to bring the body's natural defense mechanisms into proper working order, so that the liver, kidneys, cardiovascular and lymph systems can begin to work efficiently to detoxify.

In some way, this can be seen as investigating what is causing the rebellious cancer cells to revolt in a society (*the "bio-terrain"*) as meticulously co-operative as the human body, and to discover resources to alleviate their stress. By removing the uncollected garbage (*toxins*) that is filling the streets (*the lymphatic system*), and preventing the proper flow of traffic, (*blood flow*), the body's natural defense mechanism (*immune response*), is able to work efficiently again. *The "bio-terrain" is restored.*

*How do we do this?* First, stop the toxic input and gently begin to cleanse the system. Start with the kidney flush, which is an herbal formula to drink daily as a tea. Follow with a liver and gallbladder flush to remove the hundreds of small calcified stones that get built up in the bile ducts, preventing proper elimination of waste and the regular production of bile to breakdown fats.

Next, change the diet to suit your particular body type (See Part V on Ayurvedic Living). Become a vegetarian with the correct enzyme and nutritional supplements that work to provide the missing nutrients and help to alkalinize the *ph* of body. Depending upon your situation, a short juice fast may be in order. Learn about coffee enemas and Colemaboard Hydrotherapy to cleanse the colon and small intestines. This will help to efficiently remove the toxins produced by the body's resultant attempt to purify itself.

Introduce fresh squeezed vegetable juices every day. Exercise and emote. Breathe and relax. Retreat and rest. Contemplate what lessons you have to learn from this unexpected visitor. *Surrender* to a new way of living. Cooperate with the cancer messengers who are literally trying to keep the body alive, containing the aberrant cells in tumor form by accumulating the toxins that the overly taxed immune system could not handle. Let go of the old lifestyle and be active in positive ways to rejuvenate and rebuild the body's natural defenses.

For a more in depth and comprehensive treatise on the theory of cancer as a defense mechanism, please read the brilliant book *"Cancer is NOT a Disease - It is a Defense Mechanism"* by Andreas Moritz, or any of his other books on health and healing. You can visit his website at www.ener-chi.com

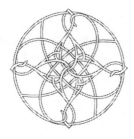

# CHAPTER 10

# THE MIND/BODY CONNECTION

*"Where the mind goes, the body must follow."*

Deepak Chopra

SINCE the groundbreaking work of Deepak Chopra's 'Quantum Healing' twenty years ago, much has been discovered and written about the connection between the body's reaction to the minds' thoughts. In this seminal book, Chopra lays out the principles of healing the body naturally, utilizing the innate defenses of the immune system, chemically linked with what the mind thinks during the healing process.

Neuropeptides are protein molecules connecting a thought and a bodily reaction. Neuropeptides and neurotransmitters, deriving from our DNA, not only come from the brain, but have been found to be part of the intelligence of the immune system. Therefore, this intelligence, sending the necessary help and information via the complex carbons, atoms, amino acids and proteins, is a major factor in governing the correct chemistry for healing the body. These neuropeptides are everywhere in the body, traveling piggyback on trillions of cells, delivering the necessary nutrients and chemicals throughout the body.

The brain and the immune system are intimately connected to one another. Indeed, we could say they are one and the same. For if we have a happy, optimistic thought about healing, the immune system instantly responds, going to work to produce the necessary peptides and leukocytes (white blood cells which are also called killer "T" cells), that will travel to the site of the disease and begin to eradicate mutant cells or invasive viruses.

It is a fact that we all have cancer cells constantly forming in the body, but our immune systems are responding tirelessly to eliminate them. So why is it that one person living a relatively healthy life succumbs to cancer at a young age, while another person, smoking and drinking and eating a poor diet, lives into their nineties? It's not necessarily to do with diet, environmental stress or good genes. A lot has to do with one's attitude towards life, and the way the mind responds to different life circumstances. What we think and feel emotionally, affects us physically.

I will give you an example of this bodily response from my own experience. Several weeks after the operations to remove the tumors from my leg, I was scheduled to have a PET scan to see if there had been any metastasis to other parts of my body. For days leading up to the review of the results with my oncologist I was in a state of high anxiety, worried about the possibility of a positive diagnosis. When I entered the doctor's office I had extremely low energy. In fact I was sure I had the beginnings of the flu, or worse, another cancer in my body. Only cancer survivors know the doubt and fear that can arise over minor symptoms in the body. An unusual pain, or a night of heavy sweating, can send the mind racing with negative thoughts of a recurrence.

I sat waiting in his office, in this state of expectant anxiety, for 15 minutes, before he entered breezily and opened the PET scan results. He studied them interminably. Then he smiled and turned to me exclaiming, "Well, you're all clear!" In that instant a tremendous relief came over me, and I left his office walking on air. I got into my car and sang at the top of my voice all the way home. Needless to say, all my flu like symptoms vanished, and I experienced super-heightened energy and elation for the next two weeks.

You can see how good and bad news can affect our emotions differently and this has a direct bearing on our health. We all know the wonderful highs that can be experienced when we fall in love. Suddenly the world seems full of positive vibrations. We can skip meals and not even notice. The body is so light and energetic that we feel young and revitalized again.

After the clear PET scan, I began to feel better each week. The following months I re-entered my old life with new vigor and the feeling of being given a reprieve from the gallows. I determined to live my life more fully and to do all those things that I had been putting off until "some day".

I made plans to travel to England to see my family and, I attended a poetry tour in Ireland, something I had always wanted to do. I took a short sea cruise, bought myself some new clothes and took friends out to dinner to celebrate my love for them. I sold my small house by the beach which was damp and moldy, and bought a bigger one on a sunny hillside. My life was a whirl. I was very busy and somewhat stressed financially, worrying if I could afford the expense of the new house.

Then, in the fall of that same year, my worst fears manifested themselves. I discovered the re-appearance of a small lump on the same knee, above the scar of the last operation. I didn't tell anyone and kept my fears to myself. It was the holiday season, I was in a new house, and anyway, it may be nothing to worry about.

After a couple of months, there was no doubt that it was a return of a cancerous tumor and it was growing at an alarming rate. I told my close friends and family and renewed my search for an alternative treatment. One thing was for sure, I wasn't going back to the hospital for an amputation. This time I was on my own.

Among the herbs and remedies that I found was a cancer salve made from the Native American recipe called Bloodroot. I had heard about it from a chance pairing with some visiting golfers. One of them had used the salve successfully to remove a skin cancer and the other had eaten small quantities for prostate cancer and lowered his PSA count. I recruited my two house mates for support and began to apply the salve to the tumor which by now, although not painful, was inflamed and about the size of a large walnut shell.

I studied a book on the subject and began to apply the salve every day. Now it became really painful as the acid in the formula began to burn down into my leg. After 14 days I had only succeeded in burning away the skin, thereby exposing the raw tumor to the air. It looked like a big, angry strawberry and I had to keep it covered with bandages and ointments to prevent any infection. I couldn't shower or bathe and the pain was intense whenever I put weight on my leg.

Now I was in despair and went back to see the oncologist. He was aghast at what I had done and urged me to get the leg amputated as soon as possible. This is your only hope, he told me. I was left with the prospect of the exposed tumor growing steadily, with the likelihood of infection a real problem.

# A WALKER OF THE SHORE

It was at this low point, contemplating my choices, that I found myself limping along the local beach one evening as the tide was going out and a beautiful sunset had begun to paint the western sky. I hardly noticed the scenery and the other people strolling along, walking their dogs. I was pondering my decision deeply and contemplating life with only one leg.

I glanced up at the dipping sun and saw the crimson clouds reflected in the glassy blue ripples on the wet sand and I began to cry. I began to sob, not just for the beauty that was happening all around me, but for the impending loss of my leg and the loss of all those things that I needed it for - golfing, running, backpacking, hiking, yoga, mountain climbing and walking the shore on a beautiful evening like this. A huge surge of energy, full of rage and sorrow, filled my body and I released myself into body shaking sobs, oblivious to the people around me. Then a new strength began to rise up in me. I determined right then and there that I would rather die than lose my leg. I would find another way. "I am a walker of the shore!" I said aloud, "I have been walking the shore since time began and I need two legs to do it!"

Many friends consoled me and urged me to amputate to save my life. They extolled the virtues of modern prosthetics. Everyone had a story about some person who had achieved amazing things with artificial legs. I know they were concerned for my health, but it was not their body that they were so cavalier about cutting up.

My spirits were very low. Here was a time when I couldn't see any light at the end of the tunnel. My mind went into constant fear and as a result I contracted a high fever. Every night was full of nightmares accompanied by heavy sweats that soaked the bed sheets so much, I had to wrap myself in bath towels to soak up the perspiration. I contemplated my death and my friends watched me lose weight and sink lower each day.

One night when I was at the very depths of hopelessness, and at a stage in my illness when I did not know if I would live or die, I decided to take a hot salt and soda bath. As I lay in the hot water with my leg hanging over the side, my body relaxed and I closed my eyes trying to calm my mind from the fear and anxiety about the impasse I had reached in my illness. Suddenly everything became very quiet like I had entered a tunnel into another universe. I found myself sitting on a horse, staring at a vast sandy plain, with magnificent colored rock formations far across the valley.

Everything was blindingly clear and the landscape was saturated with deep colors. I could feel the warm wind on my face and the hot, twitching skin and breathing body of the horse underneath me. I was aware of another person on a horse standing to my left and intuitively knew it was my dear friend Walter, who lived in my house, and had been taking care of me for weeks.

From out of nowhere in the distance we saw a Native American approaching us rapidly on a pinto horse. He was a magnificent figure with buckskin pants and eagle feathers in his hair. He carried a lance festooned with feathers and colored beads. It was as if this meeting was pre-arranged, and we were not afraid as he came to a stop in front of us, the dust kicking up and shrouding us briefly. He stared straight at me and I heard a voice in my head say distinctly, "If you find the will to live, you will not die at this time." That was it. His face was strong and impassive. He glanced briefly at Walter, wheeled his horse around, and rode off the way he had come in a cloud of dust.

Sound suddenly returned and I came out of the trance-like state with a whoosh and sat up breathlessly in the bath. That night I had a profoundly deep sleep and when I woke in the morning something had changed. I felt better. Color had returned to my face and I felt a new strength and a will to live. I sat up in bed and, with all the strength I could muster, I yelled out "I WANT TO LIVE!! I WANT TO LIVE!!' Walter came rushing up the stairs and smiled and said "Well you look much better, brother. I was worried about you there for a while."

## THE CURANDERA

I renewed my prayers for help and continued to search for a more natural cure. Then it came to me, as these things often do at the eleventh hour, by a chance referral to an angel. She was a Mexican/American Curandera or female healer and herbalist practicing in the mountains of San Bernardino County, California. This woman wild crafted and formulated her own herbal medicine, having learned the healing arts as a young girl from her grandmother in Southern Mexico.

One telephone call convinced me that I needed to visit her as soon as possible. Helene was a wealth of new information and talked a mile a minute about positive ways to help me. She didn't seem phased at all by my exposed tumor situation and told me to come and stay with her for a week. My spirits picked up and along with them my energy level. With my leg painful to walk on, I still couldn't drive a car, so I enlisted the help of Frank, a Somatic Therapist and close friend and confidant, visiting me from Switzerland. When we arrived the next week I was immediately buoyed by Helene's positive spirit. I spent each day doing a variety of treatments with regular ozone infusions to shrink the tumor.

At this time I was doing an almost raw, vegetarian diet, which I thought would purify my system, and I had lost a lot of weight. Helene insisted that this was a wrong diet for me now and entreated me to start eating meat again to build my strength back up. She was right! That lunchtime Frank and I visited a local Thai restaurant Helene had recommended. I had the best roast duck I have ever eaten in my life. I walked out of the restaurant with renewed strength, my body literally pulsating with energy.

# THE SERMON ON THE MOUNT

A little later that day Frank stopped the car at a view point which overlooked the valley of Los Angeles. From that high up, we could see nothing for miles but the tops of the San Bernardino mountain range and a giant blanket of smog covering the city. We sat and talked very intimately about the truth of my situation. I had known Frank for many years and he asked me to inquire deeply into the purpose of my life. His question stunned me and I had one of those mind stopping intuitive insights. I was as unhappy with my life as I was before the cancer. If I was given a chance to live, what would I do with my life?

I didn't have an immediate answer but I knew right then that my life had to change radically. I had to simplify everything and sell the big house that was a cause of so much financial stress. I needed to find purpose in my life!

I continued to improve and realized again the importance of positive thought and action on the healing process. I visited Helene a second time the following month and she recommended we move to plan B; remove the tumor. She worked closely with a Mexican M.D. and oncologist named Dr. Salvador Vargas. She arranged a meeting with him in Los Angeles and a few weeks later I arrived at his clinic in Tijuana.

Dr. Vargas introduced me to his surgeon, his radiologist and his wonderfully compassionate staff. They performed the tricky operation to remove the tumor successfully and it cost just $3000, a fraction of what it would cost in the US. From then on I visited Tijuana every month for low doses of chemotherapy and radiation, a treatment that Dr. Vargas has developed over 30 yrs as an oncologist.

I was fed with I.V. bags containing high doses of vitamin C and minerals, along with infusions of liquid Laetrile, the amazing cancer healer derived from apricot pits. I also was given a special anti tumor serum, made up of amino acids, called Aminex. I later administered this serum to myself, three times a week for nearly two years, through an I.V. catheter implanted into my chest, Both Laetrile and Aminex are banned by the FDA in the US.

Dr Vargas is available at the Servicios Medicos al Oncologia Integral clinic in Tijuana, Tel. 011 52 (664) 634 3298 or 011 52 (664) 634 3993 and at www.s.vargasz@yahoo.com or www.betaniawest@live.com . You can contact his assistant in the US at 1 951 232 3133 or 1 888 396 3130.

Helene Gentili is at www.info@healingrose.com She has since moved her practice to Marin County, just north of San Francisco. Helene is a true healer and superb natural herbalist.

To this day I am grateful for these healers who came to my aid when I so desperately needed it. There is no doubt that a positive attitude and a healing plan with caring providers can greatly assist the road to recovery. Medical staff can convey fear and negative emotions that will be absorbed by your deep unconscious. That is why it is now standard procedure for surgeons and operating room staff to not say anything negative during surgeries. It is believed that it can be unconsciously picked up by anesthetized patients, affecting the outcome of the operation. It is a good idea, if you must have surgery, to make a tape for yourself with your own message of positive affirmations such as:

- My body knows how to heal itself and will make a full recovery from the operation.
- The operation will be successful and remove all cancer from my body.
- My body will control the bleeding and cooperate with the surgeon.

You may add your favorite soothing music by talking to the unconscious in positive, reassuring ways, affirming one's safety, and orienting the mind to be ready to wake up from the anesthetic. Most nursing staff will be happy to make sure that your headphones are in place and the tape operating before the anesthetic takes effect.

I hope this story of my journey through cancer helps you see how important it is to keep the mind positive, thereby facilitating the bodies' healing process. Remember; always surround yourself with positive people and ideas!

# PART II

# THE BODY

*"And is it not important to realize*
*what faith does for human beings,*
*for their well being, for their healthiness*
*of soul, and — because this is also*
*the determining factor for physical health —*
*for their body too?"*
—Rudolf Steiner

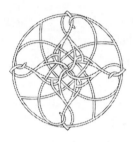

CHAPTER 11

# THE NATURAL CANCER REMEDIES

*"My advice is: Be a part time fanatic.*
*Saving the world is only a hobby.*
*Get out there and enjoy the world, your girlfriend,*
*your boyfriend, husband or wife.*
*Climb mountains, run rivers, enjoy life,*
*do whatever you want to do while you can,*
*before it's too late."*

Edward Abbey
Environmental Advocate and Author of
The Fools Progress

THE following information about alternative and natural medicine, to be used by itself, or to complement the conventional western approach to cure, was collected and tested by me over a period of several years. These are some of the cancer remedies that I feel were very effective out of many that I tried. However, what worked for me won't necessarily work for you. So which one is best for you? Use as many as possible! I believe in throwing everything at cancer to see what sticks. Don't be afraid to experiment and listen to your body's response. Finance may be a factor for you. I spent nearly all of my life savings trying different remedies and pursuing treatments out of the country. When your life is at stake, don't be a miser.

Beware the *"You need to...!"* factor. You may be inundated with friends calling you up about the latest treatment that they heard of. *"You need to see this doctor!"* or *"You need to try this treatment or read that book (or article)!"* Sometimes the influx of information can be overwhelming. Let a family member or a friend do the follow up research before you devote your time to it. Believe me, I know, you can get really aggravated by friends' well meaning intentions and the overload of information that they feel *"You have to have!"* or *"You need to do!"* Just remember it is their love and caring for you that is motivating their need to give you information.

# THE FOUR PARTS OF THE NATURAL CANCER RECOVERY PROGRAM

1. The foundation is Ayurveda and its principles of diet, daily and seasonal lifestyle practices and the emotional/spiritual awareness of the mind. All these elements are considered and applied to the particular constitution of the individual.

2. The second part is the Metabolic Medicine model for cancer patients designed by Dr William Kelly, with its emphasis on cleansing routines and enzymatic formulas to remove cancer cells from the body.

3. The third component is my own years of research and experimentation with natural detoxification and cleansing in recovering from my own cancer, and their integration with Ayurveda Pancha Karma and the long term cancer recovery program.

4. The final part is what has been termed "The New Medicine" or what I call *"soul work."* This is the underlying emotional conflict at the root cause of all disease. This emotional factor must be *re*-discovered and released for true, long lasting healing to be effective.

The next few chapters will talk about food and diet which are the mainstay of recovery and rejuvenation during and after cancer. This will be refined in the following chapters on the Ayurvedic diet and lifestyle, which I feel is the ideal combination for the prevention of disease and the continuation of a healthy way of life.

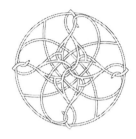

CHAPTER 12

# WHAT TO EAT?

*"In a famous study from the seventies,*
*some laboratory rats were fed a packaged breakfast cereal*
*and some were fed the cardboard box the cereal came in.*
*The rats that ate only the box lived longer."*

IT is no secret that the rise of cancer rates to epidemic proportions in the west during the last 50 years, is directly linked to the beginnings of pre-packaged and preserved food in supermarkets. Large corporate food conglomerates, interested in making more profits from a longer shelf life and less spoilage, have denatured food and laced it with preservatives. Add to this the fast food outlets, animal factory farms, hormones and growth agents in animal feed, chemical pesticides and crop fertilizers and, more recently, though not yet well studied, the use of genetically modified organisms (GMO's) to make food grow faster, bigger and be more resistant to insects. Today we have a "perfect storm" for the makings of an unhealthy population.

While environmental pollution and stressful lifestyles contribute to illness, there can be no doubt that the food we eat is a critical factor in the rise of cancer and chronic disease in the United States and other countries copying the western lifestyle and it's eating habits. The good news is that with a little discipline and discrimination, we can all eat a delicious, highly nutritious and balanced organic diet that will keep us in optimal health throughout our lifetime.

Everyone's body is entirely unique and requires a particular diet of food, water and oxygen to balance it physically and metabolically. The old saying, "you are what you eat" is only partially true, more correctly, "you are what you *digest*." This is because your body converts the nutrients and proteins it assimilates into energy, which in turn feeds the blood, bones, tissue, skin, nails, hair, etc. Consequently the more nutritious your food and the more efficiently you assimilate it, the healthier and stronger your body will grow.

It is important to realize that each person must find the right combination of nutrients for themselves whether their diet is vegan, vegetarian or includes animal products. Maybe your diet has been pretty healthy up to now, but your body is asking for a change to bring it back into balance. If you have not been very nutritionally conscious up to this point, now is the time to consider a change for the better.

There are some well known rules about diet when dealing with cancer. The very first is absolutely no sugar! Cancer cells thrive on sugars, so begin by letting this one go. Sugar comes in many forms and is hidden in a lot of processed food in the form of high fructose corn syrup (the main ingredient in sodas), fructose, sucrose, dextrose, and even more detrimentally in the chemical sweeteners like NutraSweet, Splenda, Sweet n' Low and other artificial sweeteners known to cause cancer in laboratory rats.

Once sugar is removed from the diet in these forms, it takes one or two months for the addiction to subside. Gradually your body will come more into balance. By adding good protein in the form of organic dairy products, fish and white meat; you will eventually overcome the sugar craving. Let go of the habit of eating a dessert after meals and in time when you are recovered enough you can introduce healthy sugars such as honey, maple syrup or succanat.

It is best to avoid stimulating beverages such as coffee, black tea (substitute green tea) and all forms of soda and alcohol. These are our little consolations in life and may be difficult to give up; but this is not forever, so ask yourself, "Do I really want to get well?" and make the choice. You may never go back once you begin to experience the health and vitality gained from eating a pure diet.

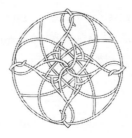

# CHAPTER 13

# THE CANCER DIET

*"At each stage of learning we must give up something, even if it is a way of life that we have always known."*

Ginevee – Australian Aboriginal.

AFTER my first cancer operation to remove the tumor I became a strict vegetarian. Six months later, I was off crutches and my leg was healing slowly although I had lost weight and my daily energy was low. I decided that what I needed to convalesce, was some sea air. So I realized one of my 'some day' wishes and booked myself on a luxury cruise ship for a 5 day trip down the California coast to Mexico and back.

The fresh sea air was invigorating and each day I would limp around the promenade deck, gradually increasing my endurance. These ships are like floating five star hotels and the multiple buffets feature a fabulous variety of food choices; all you can eat buffets for breakfast and lunch, with dinner being a sumptuous sit down five course meal offering a variety of mouthwatering meat entrées and one vegetarian dish, which I always chose to eat.

It was only the second day at sea but my energy was quite low. Around mid-afternoon I became quite fatigued. Checking in with my body I became aware that I was craving protein and I went in search of a peanut butter sandwich. The restaurants being closed, I came across one of the many snack carts, this one offering a help yourself buffet of Mexican taco fixings. Maybe some refried beans and rice would do the trick I thought and I picked up a taco shell and began to serve my self from the many fixings available. It was then that I saw the tray of hot chicken fajita strips sizzling in a bed of special sauce. It smelled delicious and my body reacted immediately. My mouth started to salivate uncontrollably and my whole body screamed "EAT CHICKEN NOW!"

Before I could help myself, I was lathering layers of chicken strips onto my taco. I didn't even wait to sit down and stuffed the taco into my mouth right there standing at the buffet cart. My body and brain began to flood with visceral pleasure and energy as I swallowed the first taco. I quickly made up two more chicken filled tacos and sat down to savor them calmly.

That night in the restaurant at dinner I splurged on the lobster and every night following I sampled a different meat entrée. I began to feel more energy each day and increased the number of times I circled the promenade deck impressively. By the end of the cruise I had added a healthy 5 pounds to my skinny frame and felt ten times better.

Some cancer survivors become strict vegetarians and profess that this saved their lives and they continue this diet for the rest of their lives. I actually recommend a detox of the system and some raw foods and vegetable juices and a vegetarian diet for a period of time after surgery and/or other treatments, to boost the body's nutrient intake. I recommend a period of at least 6 to 12 months on a vegetarian diet until the body is cleaned out and feels healthy again. During this period some fish, once or twice a week, may be appropriate for extra protein. Just make sure it is wild and not farmed fish. Include morning shakes with whey or hemp protein powder and raw soaked nuts and seeds along with nutritional and enzyme supplements and this should round out the diet for the first 6 months or so.

This works well for some people, but after a period of time the body needs building up, so after a serious illness with surgery and related treatments, you may eventually want to support your recovery with organic white meats like fish, chicken and bone broths. Once in a while add organic buffalo meat or field raised lamb depending on your taste. Your body will tell you when and if it is the right thing for you.

To eventually add meat to the diet depends entirely on your own rate of recovery and the type of cancer you are dealing with. It is a personal choice and should be subject to your health and the signals your body will give you, with your best interests in mind. Remember, at first you are attempting to flood the body with powerful phyto-nutrients, mostly from green plants, and this is the way to build a healthy immune system right from the start.

I do not recommend fasting right after a diagnosis or traditional treatment. Again it has to depend on your situation, age, time of year etc. This may be appropriate later under the supervision of a health professional when the cancer is on the run. I do recommend a serious look at your diet. If it is heavy on red meat, processed foods (anything in a packet) and sugar (especially high fructose corn syrup), it may be time to look at its implication in your loss of health.

Start with cleansing the body. Do the kidney, liver and gallbladder flushes. Introduce juicing every day and bring in more raw foods and green smoothies. Cook at home. Become vegetarian conscious and begin to rejuvenate your body with clean, nutritious food. An excellent recipe book for cancer patients is "Eat Well and Live" by Gwynn Palmer available from Sound Food Publishing, P.O. Box 4965, Clearwater, FL. 3378, USA. www.soundfood-publishing.com

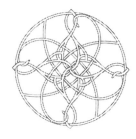

# CHAPTER 14

# NOURISHING TRADITIONS

*"Breakfast like a King, lunch like a Prince and dinner like a pauper"*
Anonymous

THE best advice I found for a general all round natural diet, comes in the book called Nourishing Traditions by Sally Fallon. Based on the fascinating research by Western A. Price, a dentist who, in the 30's and 40's, purely as a hobby of professional interest, studied the dental health of indigenous tribes worldwide, living outside the cultural norms of civilized society. Ostensibly looking for what created the healthy teeth and jawbone structure that he invariably found amongst these tribal peoples, he noticed that they all exhibited optimal health on many levels, including emotionally harmonized families and communities.

What he discovered was a diet, common to all of the diverse communities, that consisted of basic, all round, naturally occurring foods, grown, foraged and hunted locally. This included wild meat, oils from plants and nuts, wild crafted herbs, fresh fruits, whole butter and milk from livestock and, if they lived in a coastal area, a variety of sea foods. Common to all were the fresh home cooked meals that the families ate together. Not only did the people have near perfect dental and bone structure, there were no incidences of cancer or degenerative diseases and the people were invariably contented and happy.

Studying the same groups of people year after year, Price began to notice the introduction of processed and manufactured packaged foods from the west, and he saw a real decline in overall health, including tooth decay and western type diseases unknown in these cultures before.

The lesson we can take from this is to eat a balanced diet that includes oils, fats, fruits and green plant food from natural sources close to where we live. Once you introduce processed, packaged food, chemically laced to increase shelf life and profit, you are compromising the nutrition your body needs to stay optimally healthy.

Finally it should go without saying that all types of 'fast food' should be avoided. The ingredients are laced with taste enhancing chemical additives, pre-cooked, frozen, trucked in over long distances, and then cooked again in deep fried oils. This food is often eaten 'on the run' and is not digested properly. Always sit down and eat food in a relaxed atmosphere, allowing 5 minutes at the end of the meal to sit a moment before moving on to the next activity. If possible visit your local Farmers' Market or natural food store. You may pay a bit extra for organic food but your life could depend on it. You can't put a price on that.

Now let's talk about what foods specifically promote healing. Fresh food cooked at home should include leafy greens such as kale, collards, chard, mustard greens, spinach, dandelion greens, broccoli, and cabbage. These can be steamed or lightly sautéed in oil or ghee with some turmeric, ginger and mustard seeds, then add some water and simmer for several minutes. Together with steamed rice or a baked sweet potato, they make a highly nutritious combination that is easy to digest. Depending on the season and availability, fresh fruits and salads are very beneficial if your body can tolerate them. Soups containing chicken and/or root vegetables are excellent blood builders.

Eat regularly at set times with 4 to 5 hours separating meals. Don't skip meals and don't snack in between except for fruit if you are hungry. These parameters will depend on what your body can tolerate at your stage in the healing process. Trust what your body tells you and try to avoid frozen foods and the use of microwave ovens as these two things change the molecular structure and damage the nutrient content of the food.

Dr. Vargas, a my Mexican doctor, once told me his theory on the high incidence of cancer in the U.S. compared to Mexico. "What do you find in the upper kitchen cabinets of American kitchens?" he asked. To which he added, "Cheap vitamins and all sorts of canned and packaged, preservative filled food and supplements. And what will you find in the cabinets in Mexican kitchens?" he asked with a smile. "Peppers, beans, herbs and flour to make tortillas!" The Mexican diet may be quite basic but the incidence of cancer has been quite low compared to America until recent times. Amongst the new culprits this doctor mentioned were manufactured building materials of pressurized woods, plywood, pressed wood panels and synthetic carpets exuding chemicals, instead of the traditional Mexican building components of cement block, stucco and ceramic tile.

Sally Fallon's Nourishing Traditions book talks about what foods make small indigenous populations more healthy and encourages us to eat a varied diet incorporating all natural, organic food. It has many wonderful facts and recipes for you to experiment with and this may be a way of life to choose, after the initial cleansing and vegetarian diet, if you feel you need more protein in your diet. In the next chapter we will explore specific foods in detail that are known cancer fighters.

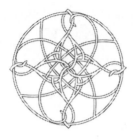

# CHAPTER 15

# CANCER FIGHTING FOODS AND RECIPES

*"Let food be thy medicine"*

Hippocrates

## JUICING

THIS is standard practice for anyone wishing to flood the body with instant nutrition. If you don't have a juicer, buy one! There are many varieties out there but the masticating, crushing, grinding types are said to preserve more of the available nutrients for absorption by the body. The centrifugal type is faster and easier to clean but may preserve less nutrient value, but whatever you choose will be a real plus for your recovery. If you are too weak to do it yourself, get help. The helper can share the juice as a reward. It is a labor intensive process, especially if you add in the regular visits to the market to get fresh organic produce, but well worth the effort. Drink two or more glasses a day for optimum benefits.

Fresh organic carrots make an excellent base, to which you can add any combination of vegetables such as beets (including their greens), celery and any of the leafy greens. Adding a lemon, a thumbnail of ginger root and an apple to the basic carrot combination is a favorite of mine. Always use organic where available otherwise you are running the risk of adding pesticides and chemical fertilizers to the mix. If organic is not available, wash the vegetables in a well diluted bleach solution and thoroughly rinse. Vegetable juice is preferred over fruit juice because it alkalinizes the system and helps balance the PH levels.

# POWER SMOOTHIES

Many people feeling unwell cannot eat a heavy meal in the morning and power smoothies are a meal in themselves and pack a real protein punch. Start with a base of Almond, Oat, Rice or Hemp milk, or just plain fruit juice such as apple. Add some combination of the following:

Power Smoothie Recipe

Put in a blender 1/1½ cups of Almond Milk, Rice Milk or Hemp Milk*

Add:

- 1 tsp green powder such as Spirulina, chlorella, blue green algae, barley grass or a green mix such as VitaMineral Green.
- 1 scoop Whey powder (pure protein), Hemp Powder (watch out for sugar content in cheaper brands!)
- ¼ cup of sugar free yoghurt.
- 1 Tbls brewers yeast.
- 2 Tsp Lecithin (keep in refrigerator)
- 1 Tbls fresh wheat germ, (keep refrigerated).
- 1 tsp Cordyceps powder. (Chinese mushroom). *Optional*
  OR
- 1 tsp Maca (South American root tonic) *Optional*
- Add any fresh berries (frozen blueberries are OK)

Of course using all of the above ingredients you will end up with a pretty potent drink and so you must decide the right combination for your digestive system.

*Much of the Soy Protein powder and soymilk is genetically engineered (GMO's) and Soy products are contra-indicated in the treatment of some hormone related cancers. With the controversy surround Tofu it is best to avoid it.

## GREEN BREAKFAST DRINK

I drink this most mornings and adapted it from a formula I found in Dr Majid Ali's books.

- Fill a quart mason jar with 16 oz filtered water.
- Add 1 teaspoon of 'Vitamineral Green' or any green powder.
- 1 scoop of vanilla Whey powder. (Protein)
- 2 Tbls granulated lecithin (Supports the liver)
- 2 Tbls freshly ground flax seed. (Helps the bowels and elimination)
- (optional- add 16 oz fresh vegetable juice.

## BEE POLLEN

Both the raw pollen and the propollis in a syrup form, are potent immune boosters with antiseptic, anti-viral and anti-oxidant properties. Take a teaspoon first thing every morning.

## BARLEY GREEN

This form of freeze-dried barley powder is a known anti cancer performer and you can take it diluted in juice or capsule form. A good source is Aim

International available on the internet or through one of their distributors. This product has many affidavits from cancer survivors extolling its virtues in support of their recovery.

The chlorophyll found in barley grass assists the oxygen carrying capacity of the blood. It is a rich source of vitamins, minerals, amino acids, beta carotene and SOD. This Superoxidase Dismutase is a super enzyme which boosts energy levels, neutralizes the most dangerous free radicals in the body and prevents the formation of cancerous cells. Take 6 tablespoons a day or 2 as a maintenance dose.

## ARCTIC COD LIVER OIL

Full of balanced omega 3 and 6 oils it is a powerful fat supplement. Use the flavored variety which is easier on the taste buds and keep refrigerated. Take 1 tablespoon, twice a day.

## GREEN TEA

The active ingredient in Green Tea, epigallocatechingallate (EGCG) suppresses angiogenisis , the increased formation of blood vessels feeding the cancer tumor. In one experiment, EGCG was administered to mice with stomach cancer. The results demonstrated that EGCG reduced tumor mass by 60%, while also reducing angiogenisis by a whopping 80% (*Life Extension Magazine, Dec.2009*)

A powerful anti-oxidant for fighting free radicals; use the organic blends along with other herbal teas at any time to replace coffee. It does contain small amounts of caffeine but the benefits for prevention and healing are well documented.

# ASIAN MUSHROOMS

Cordyceps, Reishi, and Maitake mushrooms come in powdered form and can be taken in capsules individually or as a combination of all three. They are excellent tonics and immune supporters and proven cancer fighters. Dr. Eliaz, www.EcoNugenics.com, makes a wonderful formula called MycoPhyto Complex, which is a combination of several mushrooms.

# MISO

Miso is a fermented soybean paste that makes an excellent soup for healing the body and is a good broth to drink when all other foods are unappetizing. It is a well documented fact that the people of Japan, who were affected by the nuclear bombings in 1945, had better rates of recovery and resistance to the fallout from radiation because of the Miso in their diet.

If you are undergoing radiation or chemotherapy treatments, drink a small bowl of miso soup every evening and to increase its nutrient value, add dried seaweeds such as Kombu, Wakame, Dulce or Hijiki. Any combination of these will add potent essential minerals to the mix.

## Miso Soup Recipe

In a separate bowl containing 1 cup of water add a small handful of dried seaweed cut into 1 inch pieces. Let these soak while you prepare the soup.

In a medium saucepan heat 2 tbls of Toasted Sesame oil and/or Olive oil.

To the pot add:

- ½ chopped yellow onion
- 1 medium carrot, sliced thin

- 1 cup of green or red cabbage chopped fine

  Stir and sauté the ingredients lightly for 5 mins.

- Add 4 cups of water

  Bring to a boil and simmer for 10 mins.

- Add the seaweed and soaking water

  Bring back to a boil and simmer for a further 10 mins.

Use a measuring jug to remove 1 cup of the hot soup stock from the saucepan.

- Add 2 heaping Tbls of Miso paste to the hot stock in the jug and mix with a spoon until dissolved.

Remove the pan from the heat and add the miso stock. Stir thoroughly and add tamari or salt to taste and a pinch of cayenne (optional). Let stand for 5 to 10 mins.

Serves 2-4 people.

# GHEE

Although not a known cancer fighter this is a superb medicine for the body. It is basically butter gently heated until the fat solids burn off and the resulting oil, when it solidifies can be used as a butter substitute. It is easier to digest, lowers cholesterol, lubricates the tissues and organs and contains essential minerals to feed the body.

A basic food and healing tool of Ayurvedic medicine, ghee is believed to be at the very heart of the nutritive healing process. Used for everything from flavoring and sautéing food to skin care and eye care, the alchemical qualities of good organic ghee are the building blocks of good nutrition. It has the highest flashpoint of any oil and will keep for months un-refrigerated without becoming rancid.

Use ghee wherever you would use butter or cooking oil. Spread it on toast or drop a spoonful on steamed greens. Always try to find an organic variety from your natural food store but if money is an issue, learn to make it yourself. It's quick and easy and cheaper and becomes a meditative process in itself.

# RAVEN'S GHEE RECIPE

<u>2 lbs</u> Unsalted Organic Butter

Drop the cubes of butter into a medium, thick bottomed, stainless steel 2 quart pot and melt on medium heat until liquid and bubbling. Now <u>immediately</u> turn the burner to low and let it simmer for an hour or more until the bubbling stops or slows down considerably. Move the fat that comes to the surface aside with a wooden spoon from time to time to check it and let the fat solids stay there or drop to the bottom.

Turn off the heat and let sit for ½ an hour. Pour into a quart mason jar through a wire sieve or cheesecloth. Let solidify uncovered, overnight and it's ready to use. Do not let it burn on medium heat or your ghee will turn brown. It should have a nutty flavor and end up a bright golden yellow. Thereafter, keep a tight lid on it and it does not need to be refrigerated. Making it on the full moon is highly auspicious and cooking it while Indian chanting or music plays in the kitchen is said to heighten its healing and medicinal powers and it will certainly heighten your spirit.

# KITCHEREE

This wonderful meal is a basic for anyone, anytime, and is traditionally given to people in India when they are sick or infirm. It was the basis of my healing recipes when I was recovering and I still make it at least once a week today. There are many versions using the split mung dahl and rice combination and here I give two, one lighter version for summer and a more soupy style using sprouted whole mung for the colder, winter months.

## Raven's Summer Kitcheree

Cooking time approx. 40 mins

Serves 4-6

- 3 1/2 cups water
- 1 cup white basmati rice
- ½ cup split mung dahl
- 1 ½ Tbls ghee
- 1 tsp turmeric powder
- ½ tsp brown mustard seeds
- ½ tsp cumin seeds
- ½ tsp curry powder
- ½ tsp salt
- 2 Tbls shredded coconut
- 1 pinch chili powder
- 1 pinch hing (asafoetida)

Put the water on a medium flame and bring to a boil in a separate pan

Heat the ghee on a low flame in a medium saucepan and add the cumin, mustard and turmeric. Stir and roast for two minutes.

Wash the rice and dahl in a sieve, drain, and add to the medium pot stirring the rice and dahl so they are cooked for several minutes in the spices and ghee.

Now add the boiling water to the rice and dahl so that the whole mixture bubbles and steams. Add the curry, hing, chili, coconut and salt and simmer on a low flame without a lid until all the water has evaporated and small holes start to appear in the surface of the rice.

When the water can no longer be seen in the holes place a lid on the pot, turn the flame to very low, and let simmer gently for about 10 minutes.

Remove the lid and fluff up the rice with a fork. Mixture should be light and airy. Serve with cooked veggies and chutney.

## Raven's Winter Kitcheree

Cooking time 1 hr.

Serves 6.

- 10 cups water
- 2 cups sprouted mung beans (soak one cup dry beans)
- 1 cup white basmati rice
- 1 cup chopped yams (or potatoes)
- ½ cup chopped carrots
- ½ cup chopped collard greens ( or other leafy greens)
- Thumbnail of chopped fresh ginger
- 3 cloves garlic chopped
- 1/8 tsp cayenne pepper
- 1 Tbls sea salt
- 2 Tbls ghee
- ½ tsp turmeric powder

- ½ tsp brown mustard seeds
- ½ tsp cumin seeds
- ¼ tsp coriander powder
- ¼ tsp cardamom powder
- 2 pinches hing
- 1 Tbls Braggs Amino Acids ( or 1 tsp Tamari)
- ½ cup of fresh cilantro, chopped fine.

Soak one cup of the dried mung beans over night, drain and let sit for a day or two so the sprouts are 1/8th to 1/4 inch long.

Take 2 cups of these sprouted beans and bring them to a boil in the 10 cups of water in a large saucepan. This will take about 10 minutes so be careful not to leave the kitchen during this procedure or the beans will boil over. Lower the flame and simmer for 20 minutes uncovered.

Wash the rice and add to the simmering beans along with the yams, carrots and greens. Add the salt, ginger and garlic and cover the pot. Turn the flame to low and let simmer for about 25 minutes. It should still be slightly soupy at this stage.

In a small skillet heat the ghee on a medium flame and add the cumin, turmeric, mustard seed, coriander, cardamom and hing. Heat until the seeds pop and release their flavor, then quickly add this to the large pot of rice, beans and veggies. Stir in the cayenne and Braggs, cover and let sit for 10 minutes for the flavors to mingle.

Serve in bowls with a sprinkle of freshly chopped cilantro, a squeeze of lemon and your favorite chutney.

# PESTO

Full of essential fatty acids (EFA's), Pesto is a wonderful and nutritious supplement to any dish. Serve it on crackers or bread.

Blend in a food processor

1 bunch cilantro

1 bunch basil

¼ cup organic olive oil

¼ cup pumpkin seeds (or walnuts)

2/3 cloves chopped garlic

Juice of 1 lemon

Salt and pepper to taste

# THE THREE SUPER SPICES

*"I have an earache"*
*2000 BC---Here, eat this root*
*1000 AD---That root is heathen, say this prayer*
*1850 AD---That prayer is superstitious, drink this potion*
*1940 AD---That potion is snake oil, swallow this pill*
*1985 AD---That pill is ineffective, take this anti-biotic*
*2000 AD---That anti-biotic is artificial, here, eat this root*

# TURMERIC

Although there are many herbs and spices used in the Ayurvedic medicine chest and kitchens of India, perhaps above all, the unassuming turmeric root has ascended to the top of its class as its powerful curative properties have been recently re-discovered by the West.

A native rhizome of Asia, its main ingredient is curcumin and it has been used in everyday cooking for thousands of years. It is the staple ingredient of curry and its blood-purifying properties are well documented. However, recent studies performed by established western medical institutions have found its healing powers to go much further. It has been tested and proven effective for its application to cancer patients to prevent and reverse tumor growth. It is effective in all nervous system disorders such as Parkinson's, Multiple Sclerosis and Alzheimer's. It is anti-biotic, anti-septic, anti-bacterial and anti-fungal. It is anti-inflammatory and a very powerful antioxidant helping to fight free radicals and provides DNA protection against damage by carcinogens. It is effective against skin cancers and applied to wounds, it will slow bleeding and prevent infection.

It stimulates glutathione S-transferase, a detoxifying cancer protective enzyme. It inhibits pre cancerous colon lesions and suppresses colon cancer. It inhibits leukemia at initiation, promotion and progression. It is a bitter herb and therefore it stimulates the liver making it more effective at producing bile. It is effective in the control of diabetes and several varieties of skin disease when the paste is applied topically, being used on bites, stings, bruises, wounds and rashes.

Everyday in every Indian kitchen this herb has been in use for thousands of years. Any wonder then that Alzheimer's and Parkinson's are rare in India. Although it is often prescribed in Ayurvedic herbal formulas, cooking with it is the easiest way to assimilate it into the system. It is bitter, astringent and pungent and cooking with it makes it palatable to the taste.

For cancer sufferers it is a must for everyday use. For prevention and cancer survivors, take 1 to 2 tsp in water before food in the morning. Add a dash of fresh ground black pepper which is said to increase its potency. If you are fighting cancer take 2 tsp twice a day, morning and evening. Buy the organic, bulk herbal powder, not the variety you will find in the little glass herb jar in the grocery store, which has probably been irradiated. Make it a staple in your kitchen and cook with it everyday. Sprinkle it on your food or stir fry your veggies in it. No bigger in size and shape than your finger, the little turmeric root has earned the title 'King of Herbs".

# GINGER

Second only to Turmeric in its healing powers, ginger is known as the "Universal Medicine" for it can be prescribed for any malady with some positive results. Commonly acknowledged for its digestive properties, the dried version is slightly hotter than the fresh root and is used in many Ayurvedic formulas for that purpose. The fresh ginger is grated or finely chopped and added to cooked dishes. An excellent appetite enhancer is achieved by cutting a thin slice of the fresh root and adding a sprinkle of rock salt and lime juice. Chewed and swallowed before meals it will intensify the digestive fire, increase the appetite and clean the tongue and throat.

- Ginger will relieve bloating and abdominal distention due to gas. The dried ginger is added to Pippali (long pepper) and black pepper to make a formula called Trikatu. The powder is mixed with hot water and is used to relive congestion of the lungs, coughs and colds.

- Given with Turmeric in warm milk the dry Ginger will loosen and liquefy thick respiratory congestion.

- Fresh Ginger can be sliced into pieces and boiled for a few minutes in water. Strain and pour into a cup and add honey and lemon juice for a soothing tea for sore throats and influenza symptoms. The ginger can be reused several times before it loses its potency.

It is not renowned as a cancer fighter on its own but used in everyday cooking it will improve your digestion and blood circulation and help to restore health.

# GARLIC

Garlic has been around for thousands of years and there are dozens of varieties available from your local farmers market. So accepted were its healing properties that it was used in ancient times to ward off evil spirits and was once referred to as "Beloved of the Greeks". It contains 5 of the 6 tastes in Ayurveda. The root is pungent, the leaf bitter; the stalk astringent; the tip of the stalk salty and the seed sweet.

Garlic contains allicin which destroys detrimental bacteria within the body. Diallyl sulphide is formed in the body from the conversion of allicin and may decrease the incidence of colon cancer by up to 75% and provide 100% protection against esophageal cancer.

The many other minerals this little clove contains include calcium, copper, essential oils, iron, magnesium, manganese, phosphorous, potassium, sulphur, zinc, Vitamin A, B1, B2 and Vitamin C. It enhances the immune system because of its high levels of selenium, glutathione and germanium.

It has many wonderful healing properties and is said to be an aphrodisiac. It is a blood purifier and helps lower cholesterol. It strengthens the memory, sweetens the throat, purifies the vision and improves the complexion, digestion and tissue nutrition. Other disorders it is useful for are "…..healing fractured bones, hemorrhoids, colic, worms, dry skin, cough, heart disease, chronic fevers, asthma and indigestion. It improves the appetite and the circulation and decreases high blood pressure and body and joint pain." (*Svoboda, "Ayurveda. Life, Health and Longevity"*)

In many studies garlic and onions have been found to act positively in reducing the risk of cancer and degenerative disease including heart disease, arthritis, liver disease, ulcers and skin infections.

It is a renowned panacea for any illness, and cancer survivors should consume it daily. The father of an old friend of mine who lived in Pennsylvania, planted garlic every Fall from the cloves he saved from the previous year. He ate one or two raw cloves everyday of his life and despite years of very toxic work spraying paint on the interiors of metal tanks, without any protective mask, he lived a robust life well into his nineties. You may not be able to eat it raw and heating garlic will reduce some of its healing properties so always add it toward the end of cooking or crush it and spread on garlic toast with fresh, ripe avocado.

# THE BUDWIG DIET

Here is something so easy, yet so extraordinarily successful in its curative power, you might tend to overlook it. Don't! The first thing I suggest to cancer patients whatever their diagnosis, is this simple formula. A German woman, Dr. Johanna Budwig, discovered this combination while working with cancer patients in the 50's and used it as part of a dietary regimen for 50 yrs with countless documented cures until she died at age 94 in 2003. She continued to lecture all over Europe until 1999 and was nominated for seven Nobel Prizes only to be thwarted each time by the ultra powerful medical establishment who lobbied against her.

All it involves is a combination of flax seed oil and cottage cheese. Why does it work? The absence of linoleic acids (found in flax oil) in the average American diet is responsible for the production of oxydase (lack of oxygen) which induces cancer cells to proliferate. Oxygen can be stimulated in the body by protein compounds of sulphuric content which make oils water soluble and easily assimilated by the cells. These are present in cottage cheese. The essential polyunsaturated fatty acids (EFA's) in flax oil act synergistically with the cottage cheese to deliver the oxygenated Omega 3 oil directly through the membrane of the cancer cell wall effectively causing apoptosis, or cell death.

Here's what an oncologist, Dr Dan C. Roehm, MD FACP (Fellow of the American College of Physicians), wrote in an article in 1990 in The Townsend Letter for Doctors and Patients :

> *"This diet is far and away the most successful anti-cancer diet in the World. What she (Dr. Johanna Budwig) has demonstrated to my initial disbelief but lately, to my complete satisfaction in my practice is: CANCER IS EASILY CURABLE.*
> *The treatment is dietary/lifestyle, the response is immediate, the cancer cell is weak and vulnerable; the precise bio-chemical breakdown point was identified by her in 1951 and is specifically correctable, in vitro(test tube) as well as in vivo (reality).*
> *I only wish that all my patients had a PhD in Biochemistry and Quantum Physics to enable them to see how with such consummate skill this diet was put together. It is a wonder!*
> *In 1967, Dr. Budwig broadcast the following sentence during an interview over the South German Radio Network, describing her incoming patients with failed operations and x-ray (radiation) therapy: 'Even in these cases it is possible to restore health in a few months at most, I would truly say 90% of the time'*
> *This has never been contradicted, but this knowledge has been a long time reaching this side of the ocean, hasn't it? Cancer treatment can be very simple and very successful once you know how; the cancer interests don't want you to know this.*
> *May those of you who have suffered from this disease (and I include your family and friends) forgive the miscreants who have kept this simple information from reaching you for so long.*
> *Signed Dan C' Roehm MD FACP*

## How to Eat It

Mix 2/3 of a cup of 1% or 2% fat organic cottage cheese with 6 tablespoons (or 1/3rd cup) of fresh, refrigerated flax seed oil. Mix together thoroughly by hand and add to a blender if you want a smoother mix. The oil is rather strong to the taste so you may want to add a little stevia or honey sweetener or as I do just add some blueberries, strawberries or banana to make it palatable until you get accustomed to the taste. <u>Eat this combination everyday!</u> As a delicious smoothie it can replace your breakfast or you can use it as a side dish with your main meal. If it is too strong for you, break it up into two batches i.e. 1/3 cup cottage cheese and 3 tbls flax oil.

When you are cancer free you should still eat it 2 or 3 times a week as I do as a preventative measure and to ensure the correct assimilation of EFA's. I could give you a lot more information here but it will be easier for you to google Budwig Diet on the internet and you will find many testimonials as to its effectiveness and even chat rooms of survivors who have used it successfully. The best website for information is www.healingcancernaturaly.com

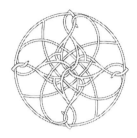

# CHAPTER 16

# CANCER HEALING HERBS AND SUPPLEMENTS

THE following is a list and description of some of the herbal treatments that I personally used and have researched. Each one contributed at some stage of my healing process and there were periods when I was using many of them simultaneously. I am a great believer in throwing everything at cancer and asking questions later. Do your own research and choose what is right for you.

## VITAMIN SUPPLEMENTS

I was recommended to try Dr. David William's Daily Advantage' as prescribed in Bill Henderson's book "Cancer Free." They come in easy traveling small packets of 8 capsules. The daily dose is two packets a day, one in the morning with breakfast and one in the evening with supper. Here's what Dr. Williams says about his nutrient package

*"I've carefully chosen the 65 vitamins, minerals, antioxidants, herbs, superfoods, amino acids and digestive enzymes that are in Daily Advantage, based on all my years of research into nutritional supplementation. These hard to find nutrients work together to supercharge the*

*antioxidants in the vitamin complex, making the overall formula more powerful and more able to destroy the free radicals attacking your cells."* I still use the maintenance dose of one packet a day even though I have a varied organic diet. Why not give your body all the nutrients you can to fight the daily pollutants in the atmosphere? They are of the highest quality and each set contains the following:

## Essential Vitamins and Minerals

| | |
|---|---|
| Vitamin A | 5,000 IU |
| Vitamin C | 2,000 mg |
| Vitamin D | 800 IU |
| Vitamin K | 60 mcg |
| Thiamine (Vitamin B1) | 50 mg |
| Riboflavin (Vitamin B2) | 50 mg |
| Niacin | 126 mg |
| Vitamin | B6 110 mg |
| Folic Acid | 400 mcg |
| Vitamin | B12 100 mcg |
| Biotin | 300 mcg |
| Pantothenic | Acid 150 mg |
| Calcium | 1,000 mg |
| Iodine | 100 mcg |
| Magnesium | 500 mg |
| Zinc | 20 mg |
| Selenium | 200 mcg |
| Copper | 2 mg |
| Manganese | 10 mg |
| Chromium | 200 mcg |
| Molybdenum | 100 mcg |
| Potassium | 100 mcg |
| Vanadium | 150 mcg |
| Choline | 100 mg |

| | |
|---|---|
| Quercitin | 50 mg |
| N-acetyl cysteine | 50 mg |
| Trace Minerals Complex | 50 mg |
| Lemon Bioflavonoids | 40 mg |
| Para-aminobenzoic acid (PABA) | 30 mg |
| Inositol | 100 mg |
| Silica | 26 mg |
| Rutin (from buckwheat) | 10 mg |
| Hesperidin (from citrus peel) | 10 mg |
| Boron | 1,000 mcg |
| Advanced Antioxidant Shield | |
| Vitamin A (as beta carotene) | 15,000 IU |
| Vitamin | E 400 IU |
| Trocotrienols (from rice) | 200 mg |
| Coenzyme | Q10 10 mg |
| Alpha-Lipoic Acid | 10 mg |
| Lutein (from marigolds) | 6 mg |
| Lycopene (from tomatoes) | 6 mg |
| Herbal Superfood Booster | |
| Spirulina (from algae) | 750 mg |
| Turmeric (from root) | 200 mg |
| L-Taurine | 200 mg |
| Siberian Ginseng Root | 180 mg |
| Bee Pollen | 100 mg |
| L-Carnatine | 100 mg |
| Royal Jelly | 50 mg |
| Astragalus (from leaf) | 50 mg |
| Ginger Root | 50 mg |
| Gymnema Silvestre | 50 mg |
| Pancreatine | 50 mg |
| Ox bile | 50 mg |
| Green Tea Extract | 50 mg |
| Siberian Ginseng Extract | 50 mg |
| Panax Ginseng Extract | 40 mg |

| | |
|---|---|
| Betaine Hydrochloride (HCL) | 20 mg |
| Ginko Biloba | 10 mg |
| Lipase | 10 mg |
| Maltase | 10 mg |
| Protease | 10 mg |
| Amylase | 10 mg |

EFA's

| | |
|---|---|
| EPA (Eicosapertaenoic Acid) | 100 mg |
| DHA (Docosahexaenoic Acid) | 150 mg |
| Other Omega-3 Fatty Acids | 50 mg |
| Gamma Linolenic Acid | 50 mg |

If this list doesn't impress you take a look at other 'multi' vitamin products available in your local health food store which often come in hard to swallow and digest 'horse' pills. In the current health food craze there is a common saying amongst nutritionists that Americans have the most expensive urine in the world. It is believed that much of the vitamins are hard to absorb and therefore expelled in the urine. This depends on the quality and metabolic structure of the product. Dr Williams has spent years formulating these vitamins and I believe they are the best you can buy. You can get more information at his website www.drdavidwilliams.com

## Vitamin D

Vitamin D is not really a vitamin, it is a hormone known as calcitrol, the most potent steroidial hormone in the body, and for years it was thought to only affect the bones by re-supplying calcium. It is now known to be a potent cancer fighter while it also affects neuro-muscular function, blood pressure, bone density and influenza.

Research has found the obvious correlation between sun exposure in the southern and western states of the US and the remarkably lower incidence of ALL cancers. Compare this to the much higher incidence of ALL cancers in the northern and eastern United States where winter months without sun prevail longer. In Northern climates the studies show 87% of people are deficient in Vitamin D during the winter months.

During the spring, summer and early fall months the UVB rays are strongest during 10 am to 2 pm and 15 minutes of daily direct sunlight on 40% of unprotected skin during these hours will be enough to manufacture about 10,000 – 20,000 IU's of Vitamin D3.

For years the application of increasingly high PF levels of sunscreen has been preventing the beneficial UBV rays from entering the body and letting in the bad UVA rays which are more harmful. It is the UBV rays that convert the cholesterol (7-dehydrocholesterol) on the skin into D3 (cholecalciferol). Even with melanoma, the deadly form of skin cancer, studies suggest the cause may be, in fact, a deficiency of sunlight; the real risk being when the skin is burned through over-exposure.

4,000 IU's of Vitamin D per day is recommended for prevention and 5/10,000 IU's per day in the winter and for cancer recovery. Take the 25 hydroxyvitamin D Test to find out if you are deficient. You can take it with a home test kit available online or through a local lab test with a blood sample. 50-60 ng/ml of serum hydroxyvitamin D levels are recommended. It has been shown in recent studies that this level results in an annual 67-70% reduction in the incidences of breast and colon cancers, type 1 Diabetes and Multiple Sclerosis within 5 years and reduces the re-occurrence rate by 50%.

Vitamin D deficiency has been linked to 17 different types of cancer and high levels of Vitamin D in the body can restore natural intercellular junctions and slow or prevent cancer growth. See the "D-Action" video and study results at www.grassrootshealth.net

# Iodine

The World Health Organization has estimated 72% of the world population is iodine deficient. This deficiency has been linked to breast cancer, prostate cancer, ovarian cysts, fibromyalgia, fibroid tumors and especially thyroid disease.

Iodized salt was introduced in 1924 to treat the high incidence of goiter disease linked to iodine thyroid deficiency but in recent years after the scare about too much salt in the diet and the switch by health conscious people to sea salt, thyroid deficiency and goiter are making a comeback along with the rise in breast and prostate cancers,

Ours soils are depleted of iodine. Chemicals in our environment such as chlorine, chloride and fluoride and heavy metals compete with the iodine receptors in our body. 25% of vegetarians and 80% of vegans are iodine deficient and have problems of thyroid disease because their diet restricts meat and dairy. Iodine rich foods include sea vegetables, cereal, dairy, fish ( cod, sea bass, haddock, perch ), meat and poultry, eggs, bread and beans.

Japan has the lowest incidence of breast cancer, prostate cancer and thyroid disease and their daily intake is 100 X more than the US. Iodine was first used in the 1800's as an anti-biotic, so if your iodine levels are low your immune system is compromised. If you have cancer start taking 50 mls a day for 3 months then drop to a maintenance dose of 12 mls a day

In breast cancer iodine helps the genes become resistant to unwanted estrogen uptake by balancing the three major estrogens and decreasing harmful estradiol making cancer prevention more effective while also increasing apoptosis ( cell death ) of cancer cells.

Iodine thins bile, stimulates lymphatic drainage and supports cellular metabolism in breast glands. These can become congested and lay fibrous tissue. The circulation is compromised, and when the blood and lymph are not flowing properly, it causes breast lumps, ovarian cysts and fibroid tumors. Fibromyalgia is caused by sluggish lymph. Cold hands, cold feet, constipation and joint pain are an indication of iodine deficiency.

## Test Yourself

The 24 Hour Urinary Iodine Load Test is the most reliable lab test which can be done by collecting urine for a 24 hr period after taking 50 ml of iodine and sending it to a lab for evaluation. There is also a quick Spot Test that can be done at home by purchasing 2% Iodine Tincture from the first aid section of your local grocery store. Dip a Q-tip in the solution and paint a 2' square on the inside of your forearm after showering in the morning. Observe it over the next 24 hours. If it disappears in less than 12 hrs it means the body has absorbed it for its use and could mean you are deficient. In this case do the 24 Hr Load Test with a lab for an accurate evaluation.

If you have been diagnosed with cancer begin taking 50 ml a day. Iodoral from www.lifespa.com is a sea vegetable blend with Bladderwack and comes in 12 ml capsules. My choice; Nascent Liquid Iodine www.magneticclay.com 4/5 drops in a cup of water every day. You want to do everything you can to increase your immune response by detoxifying the body with an efficient lymph system and good circulation. If the thyroid is fully iodized this will happen naturally.

## Additional Nutritional Supplements

In addition to a multi vitamin package I rcommend the following daily additions if your budget will afford them:

## Vitamins

| | |
|---|---|
| Vit. C | 4000 to 6000 mg |
| Vit E | 600 IU |
| Vit A | 10000 IU |
| Vit B12 | 3000 mcg |
| Vit K | 1 to 10 mg |

## Minerals

| | |
|---|---|
| Magnesium | 2000 mg |
| Potassium | 600 mg |
| Zinc | 50 mg |
| Selenium | 400 mcg |

## Supplements

| | |
|---|---|
| Glutathione | 800 mg |
| N-acetylcysteine | 800 mg |
| MSM | 1500 mg |
| Coenzyme Q10 | 1000 mg |

Digestive Enzyme Complex (incl. Chymotrypsin, proteas, lipase, papain etc.)

# VITAMIN THERAPY

Vitamin Therapy is the delivery of vitamins and nutrients to the patient by way of intra-venous drip. In a good clinic a sample of the cancer patients blood is drawn and sent, via overnight FedEx, in a refrigerated container, to a clinic in Greece where a specialist laboratory analyses it for the presence of cancer cells. If these are found in more than the normal amount, a number of tests are performed by exposing the cancerous cells to 36 different substances. Some of these are chemotherapy drugs and some are various vitamins, minerals, herbs and plant materials all known to have an effect on cancer cells causing cell death or apoptosis.

A complex report is issued stating the most effective tests and the percentage of cell death caused by each substance. A comprehensive treatment plan can then be devised incorporating some of the more aggressive elements to be delivered to the body via I.V. drip infusion.

This Vitamin Therapy (sometimes called Chelation when pulling heavy metals from the body), combines very high doses of Vitamin C (up to 75 grams), in a potent, synergistic combination with Vitamin K (7.5 grams) along with mineral supplements and the most effective of the substances found to destroy the cancer cells.

You would think a blood test telling you which chemotherapy drugs and vitamins destroyed your cancer would be readily available in the U.S. but as far as I know it isn't. The test available from the Greek Lab requires a sympathetic M.D. to order and interpret it and an alternative clinic to administer the treatments. Search for one in your area. They are out there these days but more often than not they keep a low profile because the American Medical Association (AMA) can prohibit treatment and threaten to close the clinics and cancel the licenses of the M.D. involved.

## PADMA BASIC

Some good friends told me of a DVD they had seen about Tibetan Medicine called 'The Knowledge of Healing'. They encouraged me to view it because it showed local people in the Himalayas without resource to Western Medicine who were being healed of cancer with ancient, natural healing methods. One part of this documentary shows how a combination of Tibetan herbs called Padma was proven by medical scientists in Switzerland to prevent metastasis of cancer by sealing off healthy blood cells.

While the suppliers of this formula in California do not make this claim, it is touted for its cardiovascular and immune system support and its anti-inflammatory and anti-oxidant properties. I had a lot on my plate at the time but those good friends of mine continued to research for me and found that it was available from a clinic called Amitabha, near where I lived.

The clinic in Sebastopol, California, treats many forms of degenerative diseases including cancer with Complimentary and Alternative Medicine (CAM). It has a manufacturing facility which produces high quality nutraceuticals including Padma Basic, PectaSol, Artimesinin and Mushroom Combinations, all available from www.econeugenics.com A Basic Health Guide about Padma written by Nan Kathryn Fuchs, is available from Basic Health Publications. 1-800-575-8890.

# BLOODROOT or BLACK SALVE

This herbal root, found in the southern United States, has been used by Native Americans for hundreds of years. Its power to heal cancer is still speculative but there are many anecdotal reports of its successful use in the form of a salve applied externally to minor tumors and skin cancers. Based on my own experience of applying it to the large tumor on my knee, some caution must be advised. In the special formula that includes an acid catalyst, I only succeeded in burning away the outer layer of skin and the tumor was unaffected. I have seen friends use it successfully in cases of skin cancers though, and I would recommend buying the book by Ingrid Naiman called 'Cancer Salves' which is very comprehensive and gives a good history of its use and application.

I can report positively on the use of a bloodroot formula called Vitae Elixxir in the form of a paste that can be taken internally in capsules and a tincture that is diluted in fruit juice. This special formula was developed by an interesting gentleman from Wyoming over 20 years ago. He had been diagnosed with several cancers and serious debilities. He spent many years and a lot of his own money paying some scientists to test his theories and came up with the Vitae Elixxir herbal formula. Consequently he cured himself of all the cancer. When last I spoke to him was approaching 87 and still going strong, promoting his formula and providing many testimonials of its power to fight all types of cancer. I used Vitae Elixxir everyday for over a year during my recovery and I believe it has a potent ability to heal and stop the spread of cancer in the body. Ralph Schauss can be contacted at 307-266-5310.

# HOXEY TONIC

Harry Hoxey came across an old Native American healer in the 1950's who was using an herbal formula that had been known amongst tribes in the southern United States for centuries. Containing local plants and roots, it had claims of being a cure for cancer. He opened his own clinic and began to treat patients with remarkable success. He apparently tweaked the formula slightly and would never reveal the true combination but analysts have since determined the precise amounts and ingredients.

After opening several other clinics in surrounding states and drawing an increasingly large number of cancer patients, many of them in the late stages of disease, and getting a high rate of cure, he drew the attention of the American Medical Association who accused him of practicing medicine without a license and took him to court where a long, drawn out battle ensued.

Ultimately so many successfully cured patients testified in his defense, coupled with the fact that he was asked to help one of the judges close relatives, who also had cancer, the charges were dismissed. His clinics were under constant harassment from the authorities however, so he moved his main clinic to Tijuana, Mexico where it still operates successfully to this day nearly 60 years later.

It is called the Biomedical Clinic and I visited there in 2006 for treatment. I met many returning clients who all had a story to tell and swore by the results of the tonic. I was thoroughly examined by the competent doctors and began taking the tonic daily for the next year. The herbal ingredients are all known cancer fighters and the unique combination is a powerful tool against cancer or use as a general tonic and boost to the health of the system.

# CHINESE HERBS

Chinese Traditional Medicine (TCM), while not having a track record of treating cancer specifically, should not be overlooked for bringing the body back into balance during recovery. Indeed, there are practitioners who deal with cancer specifically and I found my own Chinese doctor who made special trips to China every year to bring back the unique herbs for treatment. These herbs are boiled in a special clay pot and are taken every day. I took them for 6 months, twice a day and it was quite labor intensive to prepare them, but I do believe they contributed to my recovery.

These doctors also use acupuncture, the ancient art of using very fine needles inserted lightly into the various points on the body, corresponding to the hundreds of energy points on the meridian lines. A skilled practitioner can remove energy blocks, relieve pain and re-energize the body by knowing where to place the needles. Make your enquiries for an acupuncturist in your own area and ask if they have experience treating cancer. In Palo Alto, Northern California, contact Dr Ken Pang, 650-858-0706.

# ESSIAC TEA

Essiac tea first came to the publics notice in the 1920's when an old Native American herbal formula came into the hands of a nurse called Rene Caisse. in Ontario, Canada. She claimed that it had been prescribed to her by a woman who had been healed of breast cancer by an Ojibwa Medicine Man. At the time Ms Caisse's Aunt was dying of cancer and she decided to test the formula on her. The result was that her Aunt went on to live another 21 years and eventually died of natural causes.

Since then and up until her death in 1978 Nurse Caisse administered the herbal formula without charging for her services. She made it into a tea and called it Essiac, (her name spelled backwards) which she gave to thousands of cancer sufferers and many people have praised its effectiveness. It is believed to eliminate tumors and reduce the pain and suffering of conventional treatments. It is an excellent immune booster and liver tonic.

The modern day formula contains Burdock Root, Sheep Sorrel, Turkish Rhubarb Root, Red Clover, Watercress, Blessed Thistle, Kelp and Slippery Elm Bark. It helps relieve arthritis, prostate irregularities, urinary tract infections, circulatory problems and asthma. It can be obtained through a good herb store and the tea should be taken 3 to 6 times a day.

# YARROW

I believe Yarrow is a potent cancer fighter and I drank an infusion of it every morning. I would go into my garden where it grew profusely and clip some of its fern-like leaves, then steep them in hot water, and drink the tea. First thing in the morning and last thing at night before bed, I would squirt a dropper full of the tincture on my tongue and swallow it.

Old herbal texts referred to it as "cure of all ills". It has a potent blood cleansing ability and can remove toxins from the body. It is astringent and stops internal bleeding. It is excellent for coughs, colds and fevers and, although it is not a documented cancer fighter, I believe it is an essential herb for detoxifying the blood and can help specifically with lung diseases.

# HUCKLE IMMUNE TEA

This tea is named after a good friend, Acupuncturist and Herbalist Darren Huckle of Santa Cruz, California, who made up this blend of Chinese Herbs to help me strengthen my Qi (vital bodily energy), in my cancer recovery process. It contains four powerful herbal extracts; Astragalus, Ligustrum Berry, Eluthro Siberian Ginseng and Gymnostemma. Blend equal parts of each and add a teaspoon to a cup of hot water and drink each morning before breakfast.

# CASTOR OIL

This little bean has been used in healing for centuries. It is an annual plant that grows to 10 to 20 feet in India, South America and Asia. It is a member of the Euphorbia family and produces a light yellow oil which is non toxic and biodegradable. It is anti inflammatory and effective in malignant disorders.

Pour some on a cheese cloth and place the soaked cloth on the abdomen or an area where there is a tumor. Cover with a piece of wax paper and place a heating pad on low over it. Rest for 20 to 30 minutes.

# HYDROGEN PEROXIDE

Hydrogen Peroxide H2O2 is an excellent oxidative supplement and it's main function as a molecule is to improve the oxygenation of the body. It will improve circulation, cleanse and increase the efficiency of the lymph and blood systems, improve the capacity of the immune function and improve oxygenation of the tissues.

It will help control inflammation, prevent cancer growth and spread. It acts as an anti-oxidant, controlling the spread of free radicals by supporting the function of enzymes in the body. Best of all it is cheap and readily available at your local drug store.

I do not recommend drinking it in any diluted form. The best application is through drip infusions from a certified clinical practitioner at a health clinic near you. I recommend these weekly along with the supplementation of multi-minerals and vitamins.

At home you can do Peroxide foot soaks which help to oxygenate the tissues and eliminate toxins. This helps with inflammation and joint problems too. You can soak hands or feet or take a whole body bath.

For a 20 minute foot soak pour 10 parts warm water into a basin and add 1 part 3% Hydrogen Peroxide and 1 tsp of sea salt. Increase the ratio for a bath but in general do not add more than a 16 oz bottle to the bath water. Castor oil can be rubbed on the soaked parts after drying.

## Banned in the US and Only Available in Mexico

## LIQUID LAETRILE

Laetrile is a glucosidase also known as B17. Available in the seeds and pits of fruits and some nuts and, most commonly, in the seeds of apricots, it has become controversial in recent years. There has been much mis-information spread about it by the orthodox medical community who cannot patent it or make a profit from its sale.

I first received it when I was being treated in Tijuana, Mexico by Dr. Vargas and it is used in many of the Alternative Cancer Treatment Clinics there. For the best effect it should be taken intravenously under supervision of a medical professional. Why? Because it is more effective if given intravenously along with other vitamins and minerals such as Vitamin C and K, manganese, potassium and zinc.

This kind of Vitamin Therapy, or the intravenous injection of high doses of vitamins and minerals, is also available at Alternative Clinics in the US but you won't find high potency liquid Laetrile because it is banned in the US by the FDA. Sound familiar? The best book on Laetrile is "World Without Cancer" by G Edward Griffin in which he records the history and subsequent suppression of Leatrile and documents the hundreds of success stories of people with cancer.

Another wonderful little book if you can find it was written by Helen M. Curran called "Apricot Power : How Laetrile Cured My Cancer" In it she documents her diagnosis of Melanoma metastasized to the liver, which American Oncologists could not treat and her subsequent journey to Mexico to find a cure with Laetrile. It was self published in 1992 fifteen years after her complete recovery when she was in her early seventies.

Laetrile is available in tablet form under the name Amigdalin and is readily available on the internet. However, it can cause nausea if taken in too large a dose because of the organic cyanide and benzaldehyde that is released by the enzyme beta-glucosidase in the stomach. Another enzyme, rhodanese, present in normal tissues but deficient in cancer cells, helps to detoxify the cyanide so that it attacks the cancerous cells and leaves the healthy cells undamaged.

It is found in bitter apple seeds when you crush them in the mouth and in apricot, cherry, peach and nectarine stones. Other more available sources are elderberries, raspberries, blackberries, currants, buckwheat, tapioca, millet, almonds, macadamias, flax seeds, lentils and mung bean sprouts (see my Winter Kitcheree recipe).

Add these foods to your diet and, if you have cancer now and cannot find a medical clinic for the intravenous Laetrile therapy, you can order the bulk organic apricot kernels from the many sources you will find online. They are the richest in B17 concentrate and are relatively inexpensive. Be careful at first and build your tolerance to them gradually. I used to grind 2 or 3 of the seeds in a small coffee grinder and sprinkle them on my oatmeal or in a smoothie. They are extremely bitter and you should increase the dose slowly until you can consume 8 to 12 a day with no side effects.

Warning! Don't go overboard! This is powerful medicine and if you begin to feel the effects of 'lysing' (detoxification) such as nausea, sweating, diarrhea, headaches etc. immediately back off on the dose and allow the symptoms to subside before continuing the next day with a smaller quantity and gradually build up again.

Again I recommend finding a source to administer the liquid laetrile intravenously and for more information read the book "World Without Cancer".

# AMINEX

This serum is a powerful combination of amino acids. The main ingredient is L-Arginine, which inhibits cellular proliferation (multiplication of cancer cells) and stimulates cancer fighting T-lymphocytes. It has the ability to block the formation of many cancers, particularly tumor growth and metastasis. It is believed to stimulate the thymus gland in its ability to promote the effectiveness of natural killer cells, thereby enhancing the immune system at the same time as detoxifying the liver.

Originally manufactured in Southern California under the name Tumorix, it was banned by the FDA in the early 90's and production moved to Tijuana, Mexico, where it is manufactured under the name of Aminex. As a liquid blended serum it has to be taken intravenously and I was treated with it at Dr Vargas's clinic. While there, I was fitted with a 'pick-line' in my chest so that I could self administer it at home, twice a week for a period of 20 months. This was quite a rigorous home discipline and not cheap, (each dose costs about $50), but I sincerely believe that, along with the other treatments, it contributed to the suppression of the tumor cells in my body.

# ADDITIONAL TREATMENTS

The following are what I consider experimental supplements in the treatment of the cancer patient. Although I did not discover these until later research for this book, I would not hesitate to use them myself or suggest them for my friends and family if the need ever arose again. Please do your own research and make your own decisions.

## Protocel

After reading extensively about this treatment, my choice for the No. 1 addition for any case of cancer would be to explore the possibility of using Protocel, with the following caveat; there are many restrictions to the diet and supplementation of the patient when you use this treatment.

Developed by a chemist, James Sheridan over many painstaking years, his original formula has been copied and changed several times.

Although Sheridan was a researcher at the Michigan Cancer Center in the 1930's, he was not a medical doctor. Sheridan theorized the possibility of chemically controlling the energy needed by the cells of our body to cause energy-low cancer cells to revert to a state where the body can eliminate them as foreign matter.

The theory postulates that cancer cells are too low in energy to proceed with their normal development and the cells stop their development just short of differentiating into a normal liver, lung or brain cell and become malignant. Sheridan proposed to push cancer cells backward in their development instead of trying to encourage them to differentiate as many cancer cells attempt to do.

You can find a definitive treatise on this cancer fighter and many affidavits of its use in a great book called "Outsmart Your Cancer" by Tanya Pierce or go to the website where you can download chapters on Protocel at www. OutsmartYourCancer.com

Paul Winter's excellent website www.alternativecancer.us/protocel is loaded with information about the history, success rates, which formula to use and other protocols to avoid when taking Protocel, plus what you need to think about before deciding to take it.

# Graviola

Graviola is a natural plant drug from the seeds and leaves of a tree found in the Amazon rain forest. It has the ability to inhibit the production of ATP, the chief energy carrying compound in the body. This eventually pulls the plug on the malignant cancer cells that need huge amounts of additional energy to mutate while leaving normal cells healthy. By messing with their energy supply the malignant cells die off. Graviola is fairly inexpensive and easy to obtain and take. Studies over the last 30 years have shown Graviola to be more potent than the common cytotoxic chemotherapy drug Adriamycin and will selectively target cells from breast, colon, prostrate, pancreatic and lung.

For several years one of the big pharmaceutical companies tried to develop a synthetic version of Graviola's anti-cancer properties and failed. They knew that its natural compounds were 10,000 times more toxic to colon cancer cells than a common chemo drug. They tried to make their scientific discoveries secret, but lab results leaked out and Graviola has come to the attention of the alternative community in recent years as a potent anti tumor drug and a natural booster of the immune system. When cancerous tumors are targeted they will die off and flood the body with toxins causing weakness, nausea, headaches and aches and pains so it is important to increase the dose gradually and do colon flushes regularly and enemas everyday.

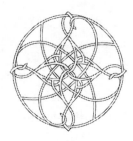

# CHAPTER 17

# DETOXIFICATION-
# CLEANSING THE BODY

THERE is no doubt that if you have a cancer diagnosis, the body is holding onto some toxic material both physical and mental. Cleansing is the <u>Number 1</u> order of business. Depending on the stage of the disease and your energy level you can begin to clear out this unwanted material that is preventing the immune, lymph, renal and cardiovascular systems from performing their efficient cleansing duties.

If you have been a consistent meat eater or junk/fast food lover, the need for cleansing is more urgent but is best done with the guidance of a health professional. While any cleansing is good for the system, if you are not familiar with the process, you may make yourself worse if you proceed too fast. It will depend on the cancer prognosis, your age, energy level and constitution.

Enemas, flushes and fasts are ways of purifying the body, and ridding it of disease. They have been used in all cultures for centuries, so while I list here some beneficial cleanses, it will have to be determined what is appropriate in your unique case.

## Enemas

This is safe to do any time and is a great way to begin to clean out the accumulated debris that gathers in the intestines over many years. The large gut that you see on many western bodies is an accumulation of intestinal fecal matter and undigested toxic waste that has turned to fat.

Enemas are best done in the morning before food intake and preferably after an early evacuation. They can be done at any time of the day or night and at least once a day for serious cases and once a week for maintenance.

Buy the required enema equipment, a hot water bottle type or better still, a plastic bucket type. Use 2 cups of warm water to begin with, temperate to the touch, and slowly build up to 4 cups (1 quart.) To this you may add herbs while it is heating such as nettle, burdock or chamomile, or steep a few green tea bags in the enema water.

An alternative is to boil a few strips of kombu (kelp) seaweed for 5 or 10 minutes in 1 quart of filtered water, turn off the heat and allow to steep overnight. Throw out the kombu in the morning and reheat the remaining water to body temperature. This seaweed enema is an excellent colon lubricant and hydrator and supplies valuable minerals to the body.

Pour the water into a glass quart measuring jug and carry it to the bathroom or place where you will be doing the enema. Hang the bucket or rubber enema bag on a door handle or sit the bucket on a counter top about 3 ft above the floor.

***Important:*** First tighten the regulating clip on the tubing about 6 inches from the end of the tubing and hold the tubing in your hand while pouring the enema water into the bucket. Now take the empty quart jar and place it on the floor. Lower the tubing and release the clip allowing about half a cup to pour into the jar before tightening the clip again. This releases any air bubbles in the tube. Pour the half cup of water back into the enema container.

Place some towels on the floor underneath yourself to catch any drips and use a pillow for your head. The more comfortable you can make yourself the easier it will be to do this regularly. Rub a little massage oil or lubricating gel on the catheter and massage the oil on your anus to make the tubing easier to insert. Cover yourself with a blanket if you wish but stay warm and play some soothing music.

Lay on your left side and bring your right knee up toward your chest as far as is comfortable and keep your left leg straight. Unclench your jaw, open your mouth and breathe deeply. Insert the catheter into your anus slowly about 6 inches. Make sure the water is the right temperature, warm but not too hot. Let the water in by releasing the clip on the tubing which regulates the flow. If the pressure builds too quickly and you feel uncomfortable, stop the flow by clipping the tube again until you feel ready to let more in. In time you will be able to allow a full quart to empty into the colon all at once. This takes about a half to one minute. When the bag or bucket is empty you will hear a slight suction sound from the container. Clip the tubing again and withdraw the tubing slowly.

Stay on your left side for a few minutes and then turn onto your back. Bring your knees up and keep your feet flat on the floor. If you are feeling adventurous you can press down with your legs and lift your pelvis off the floor to allow the water to penetrate deeper in the colon with gravity helping for about 15 seconds.

Stay on your back for 5 minutes then turn onto your right side for 5 minutes more, or up to a combined total of 15 minutes from the time you finished draining the bag. With practice you can also begin to massage the abdomen moving your hand up the left side of your abdomen and across the top of the belly toward the right side following the line of the transverse colon.

If you feel a sudden urge to release the fluid, clench the anal sphincter muscle and breathe quickly in and out for a few seconds through pursed lips. This will help you hold the solution in the colon for a few minutes more. Five, ten or fifteen minutes is ideal, but start slowly at first. You may only be able to hold it for a minute or less in the beginning but with practice you will get better at retaining it for longer periods. Eventually you will be able to do it in a more comfortable setting such as your bedroom and be able to walk to the bathroom to release the water when you feel ready.

Afterwards remember to hydrate and drink plenty of water through out the day. You will feel lighter and cleaner as you begin to flush out years of accumulated waste lodged in the colon walls. Read "Colon Health" by Norman W. Walker. His premise, and one I truly believe, is that true health begins with a healthy colon.

## The Coffee Enema

Coffee enemas date back to the early 20th century and were on the official medical guidelines for doctors until the 1950's. Along with enzymes, they are an integral part of the Daily Cancer Recovery Program because of the additional benefit of stimulating the liver to release toxic wastes along with destroyed cancer cells. The caffeine also stimulates the peristaltic muscle to help loosen encrusted feces stuck to the colon wall. Take it early in the morning so the stimulating effect of the caffeine will not keep you awake at night.

Use 3 to 4 tablespoons of organic therapy coffee available from www.s.a.Wilson.com in 1 quart of filtered water. Bring to a boil for a few minutes and turn down the heat to low and simmer for 10 to 15 minutes. Turn off the heat and allow it to cool to body temperature or make it the night before and re-heat it in the morning after straining off the grounds. You may end up with 3 cups, to which you can add another cup of water. If a quart is difficult for you to hold for 15 minutes, start with 2 tablespoons of coffee to 2 cups of the filtered water. You will gradually build up a capacity to do more.

When the urge to evacuate arises prematurely, squeeze the anal sphincter and practice breathing in and out through the mouth quickly by making a pucker shape with the lips while contracting and releasing the abdomen. The urge to evacuate will pass until the next urge comes. Laying on the right side will help retention.

## CAUTION:

The Coffee Caveat: This enema is very effective in the beginning for cancer patients who are combining it with metabolic enzymes but it is very stimulating and long term use may not be suited to your condition. Be sure to work with a qualified practitioner of Ayurveda or other Natural Medicine. Some cancer survivors still do a coffee enema every morning and feel great. How long you do it will depend on your particular situation and the program for recovery you have chosen. Coffee is a diuretic and you may find yourself needing to urinate more often.

# THE KIDNEY FLUSH

This should ideally be done prior to the liver flush, but best to begin as soon as possible in your recovery program. The kidneys are major blood purifying organs. They regulate electrolytes and maintain the acid-base balance. They receive impurities such as urea and ammonium from the lymph and blood and deposit them in the urinary bladder for elimination.

Kidney stones can form in the urethra channels leading to blockages and intense pain. Diet is the main cause of kidney stones and kidney sand. If you pull the skin just below your eyes toward your ears you may feel the presence of small lumps, pimples or coarseness which are the tell tale signs of stones in the kidneys. Buy the Kidney tea herbs from a good health or herb store and make the following tea.

## Kidney Tea Recipe

Marjoram (1 oz)

Cat's Claw (1 oz)

Comfrey Root (1 oz)

Fennel Seed (2 oz)

Chicory herb (2 oz)

Uva ursi (2 oz)

Hydrangea root (2 oz)

Gravel root (2 oz)

Marshmallow root (2 oz)

Golden rod herb (2 0z)

Directions:

Take 1 ounce each of the first three herbs and 2 ounces each of the rest of the herbs and thoroughly mix them together. Keep them in an airtight container. You may put them in the refrigerator. Before bedtime, soak 3 tablespoons of the mixture in two cups of filtered water, cover it and leave it covered overnight. The following morning bring the concoction to a boil; then strain it. If you forgot to soak the herbs in the evening, boil the mixture in the morning, and simmer for 5 to 10 minutes before straining.

Drink a few sips at a time in six to eight portions throughout the day. The tea can be drunk warm or hot but do not refrigerate it. Wait at least an hour after eating before taking your next sips. Repeat this procedure for 20 days. Be sure to also drink your 6 to 8 glasses of water each day. If you are doing liver cleanses, do a kidney cleanse every 3 or 4 liver cleanses.

If the kidney area becomes tender during the flush or the urine is a darker, brownish color, this is just the excess sand and stones being released with the herbs and you should increase your water intake at this time and add the juice of a lemon to it each day. As a benefit you may find that your sleep improves and the need to urinate at night is greatly reduced. This is because the rejuvenated kidneys are now more efficient and are filtering beneficial nutrients and re-introducing them into the bloodstream for re-absorption, instead of dumping everything into the bladder because they were too tired and weak to do their job properly. Any dark skin or pimples and bumps under the eyes will slowly disappear and your eyes and general complexion will be clearer.

The information about the liver and kidney cleanses are from Andreas Moritz's book '*The Liver and Gallbladder Miracle Cleanse*'. I highly recommend it for more information on the correct procedures for any of the cleanses mentioned here. The website is www.ener-chi.com

# THE LIVER FLUSH

*"How long will you live?*
*It depends on the liver"*

Grandma Dee Dee

The liver is probably the most important detoxification organ, keeping the heart, lungs, kidney and pancreas free from disease if it is functioning properly. It processes chemicals, drugs, alcohol, poisons, preservatives, and artificial substances and helps to eliminate them from the body.

Its functions include metabolizing essential fats, synthesizing necessary blood proteins, metabolizing and eliminating poisons and generating bile for digestion which it shuttles to the gall bladder for storage and timed release into the small intestines to emulsify fats for proper absorption.

Our fast lifestyle often compromises the proper functioning of the liver and, if you have cancer, the cleansing of this major detoxification organ is essential to begin the process of rebuilding a healthy system. When the liver/gall bladder bile ducts are congested with calcified cholesterol 'stones', no amount of fasting or a cleansing diet will be 100% successful. Many diseases besides cancer ensue when these organs are compromised including skin diseases such as eczema, psoriasis, dry skin, falling hair, tendonitis and poor digestion, which is the precursor to many more problems.

I recommend the Liver Flush recipe by Andreas Moritz from his book "*The Liver and Gallbladder Miracle Cleanse.*" Read this book before you do the cleanse, it will open your eyes about the number of health problems we can have because of an unhealthy liver.

Here's the routine:

- Choose a time between the full moon and the new moon. On, or closer to the new moon is best. Our bodies are more able to release fluids at this time.

- Eat no fats or animal products the week prior to the cleanse.

- Drink 1 quart (32 oz) of organic apple juice each day for six days prior to the cleanse. This will help soften the stones for easy elimination.

- Get a hydro-therapy colonic or colema a day or two before the liver flush. This will help the colon be able to expel the stones. Failing this, do a coffee enema each morning for three days before the flush.

- On the morning of the flush eat a light breakfast and a light lunch, no protein or fats, and do not consume anything after 2pm except water.

- At 6 pm add 4 tablespoons of Epsom salts to 24 ozs of filtered water and store in a glass jar. Then drink 6 oz of this solution (3/4 cup).

- At 8pm drink another 6 oz of the Epsom salt solution.

- At 9:30 pm squeeze the juice of two large organic grapefruit into a quart jar and filter out the pulp. You will need ¾ glass of juice.

- Pour ½ cup of organic extra virgin olive oil into the grapefruit juice, screw the lid on tight and shake thoroughly until the solution is well mixed.

- At 9:45/10 pm take this jar and stand beside your bed. You are going to bed now so be prepared. Do not sit down. Drink the mixture down standing beside your bed and do not take longer than five minutes. Use a straw or pinch your nose to help you swallow it. It does not taste bad. The consistency is strange but you can do it.

# LIE DOWN IMMEDIATELY!

- Use a pillow and do not move or speak for at least 20 minutes. You may feel the stones moving painlessly at this time.

- Now try to sleep. If you wake to evacuate in the night this is OK. You may feel some nausea as the gallbladder dumps bile into the system to deal with the oil which may back up into the stomach. Don't be alarmed. The nausea should pass.

- At 6/6:30am drink another ¾ glass of the Epsom Salts mixture.

- Rest, meditate and relax or do some light yoga until

- 8/8:30 am drink the last glass of the Epsom Salts

- At 10/10:30 am you can drink some juice or eat some fresh fruit and eat light food throughout he day.

- Remember to eat light foods for the next few days.


*The Results.*

You will have some watery stool eliminations in the morning after the flush. This is to be expected. If you use a colander to catch the eliminations you will find dozens or even hundreds of stones ranging in size from a pin head to a pea to an inch or more, depending on the state of your liver and gallbladder prior to the flush.

The elimination should be painless if you have prepared properly and you should feel light and happy afterward. If you have cancer, this should be the first of several flushes repeated every month until you see no more stones being ejected. Congratulations! You are doing a very powerful healing practice for your body and you will feel the benefit of it for many weeks.

## Liver Support Tea

This formula comes from the works of Dr Hulda Clark Ph.D N.D. You can purchase her book "The Cure for all Cancers.

6 parts Comfrey Root, Niphone root

6 parts White Oak bark, Tanner's Oak bark

3 parts Gravel Root, Queen of the Meadow

3 parts Jacob's Staff, Mullein herb

2 parts Licorice root

2 parts Yam root wild

2 parts Milk Thistle herb

3 parts Black Walnut Bark

3 parts Marshmallow root, White Mallow

1 part Lobelia, Bladder Pod

2 parts Skullcap, Helmet flower

2 quarts water.

Put 2 qts filtered water in a large pot. Add 1 cup of the herb mixture to the pot and stir well. Bring to a boil and turn off the heat. Cover and let sit for 6 hours. Bring to a 2$^{nd}$ boil and switch off heat. Strain into a jar and drink 2 or more cups of the infusion a day. You may add a little raw honey to taste and keep what you don't drink in the refrigerator.

# Root Canals and Mercury Fillings

The evidence that root canals can be a cause of cancer and many other diseases is documented in the book "Root Canal Cover-Up' by George Meinig, D.D.S, F.A.C.D. In it he tells of the work of Weston A. Price and 60 fellow research dentists. Their findings have been repressed by the American Dental Association since 1925. It showed that all root canals can be a haven for toxic wastes in the mouth and these are constantly poisoning the body. If you have root canals, have them checked, and if they are infected, if possible, replace them with a bridge and crown.

A Swiss study done by the Paracelsus Clinic routinely has every breast cancer patient remove all root canals before treatment for cancer is begun. They found that out of 150 breast cancer patients, 147 of them had one or more root canal teeth on the *same meridian* as their original breast cancer tumor.

Same goes with Mercury amalgam fillings. Get them removed from your mouth as soon as possible and replaced with safe non metal material. Have these oral treatments only done by a Biological Dentist who does not use amalgams and knows the safe protocols for removing these toxic reservoirs from the mouth.

# Lymphatic Drainage

The lymphatic channels are the most overlooked and important systems for filtering toxins in the body. Besides transporting nutrient rich plasma around the body, they act like sewers picking up waste and unwanted debris from every single cell and transporting it to the kidney and liver where it is filtered and redirected to the urinary system for disposal.

At many points along these channels are 'nodes' acting like small valves that open and close to help transport the waste. The larger and more commonly known of these are under the armpits and in the groin. When these nodes become overloaded and clogged with toxins, they can swell, causing pain and aching; this is a sure sign that they need to be massaged to help move the toxins out. _Important; Breast cancer patients should not do this massage until they are finished with therapy and feel that they are cancer free._

As part of the cleansing needed to heal cancer I recommend getting a lymphatic drainage massage from a professional body worker regularly. Second best or as a supplement to the massage, you can use a small tool called a 'gua-sha'. About the size of your hand, they are made of wood or jade with smooth, scalloped edges to fit over and around the contours of the body. By oiling yourself first you can rub over the blocked lymph nodes which are felt as tiny knots under the skin. Ask a professional body worker to show you how to do this and do it every day along with your morning oil massage.

To support a healthy lymph system, sip hot water every 15-20 minutes through out the day. Fill a thermos to make this practice easier. Eat red or golden beets grated, raw on salads or lightly steamed. The perfect lymph moving exercise is jumping on a small 'Rebounder' trampoline every day.

## Fasting

Unless you are an experienced 'health fast' person, it is important to get the help of a natural health practitioner when considering a fast. I do not recommend fasting for cancer patients until the cancer has been reversed and recovery is underway. The fast is best done in the Spring or Fall as a yearly, preventative clean out after the body has gained back its health. Often the cancer patient will have to build up body weight and energy with special foods so fasting will not be appropriate.

In a lot of cases equally good detoxification results can be gained by introducing raw, fresh vegetable juices and carefully monitoring the diet as recovery progresses. So be careful with this cleansing procedure because toxins can be released quite quickly into the system. If you decide it is the right time to do a fast, begin by eliminating food for one 24 hr period per week and drink plenty of water and herbal teas, or use freshly squeezed juices, and then reintroduce a light salad for the first meal the following day.

I recommend "Are You Confused", Paavo Airola's classic book on juice fasting from the 70's, and still good information today.

## Detox Baths

The following information was generously provided by Karen Miller-Youst HHP, Cleansing Ministries-Rejuvenation Center Santa Rosa Ca. www.cleansingministries.com 707-545-4569. (The italics are my additions).

Hot detox baths are a simple and luxurious way to detoxify the body. They are also very important to use as a means of preventing recent toxic exposure from being stored in the body as well as the releasing of stored toxins from the body. A detox bath is critical after chemical and radiation exposure such as pesticides, gasoline, dental exams, x-rays, too much sun etc. As this will support the body to quickly detox and release toxins before being stored in the tissues, it is highly recommended to take hot detox baths after massages, acupuncture, microcurrent, chelaton, fasting, aerobic exercise etc. *For any one suffering from cancer this is a way to help cleanse old toxins stored deep inside the cells for years.*

Water can only pull a limited amount of toxins by osmosis. When your body wants to release more and cannot due to toxic saturation of the bath water, it becomes overwhelmed. If you are not feeling well or are unsure of the toxoc load you will release, it is wise to start with a 15 minute bath and evaluate how you feel. If very toxic, repeat the process 12 hours later. *Cancer patients may feel unwell with an increase in heart beat and profuse sweating. This is because the water is becoming saturated with toxins and can no longer pull anymore from the body. In this case draw another bath and aim to stay in it for up to an hour until you feel relaxed and comfortable at the end of an hour.*

As with any cleanse, it is very important to be well hydrated to support the process and lessen any potential detox symptoms. Karen drinks water with lemon juice and then rubs the lemons on her skin while in the bath. Rubbing your skin with the oil and juice of the lemons ( or lemon essential oil) assists with exfoliation and the detox process.

When finished with a detox bath, you should feel tired, sleepy, relaxed, relieved, etc. If symptoms of exertion occur, empty the tub and rinse your body with cool water, If still feeling exertion, some will start over with same or different additives and feel relief after a second bath. Brain fog will usually leave after taking a detox bath. If brain fog returns you probably need to take more baths at that time.

The basic formula draws out most heavy metals and chemicals. You need the combination to get the different valences of heavy metals as each draws out different metals and chemicals.

## Detox Bath Ingredients

1 cup Apple Cider Vinegar.

1 cup Epsom salt ( Magnesium sulfate)

2 – 32 oz bottles of 3% Hydrogen Peroxide.

Adding 1 cup of baking soda can draw out radiation from x-rays, cell phone towers, computer screens, televisions, flying in airplanes etc. Running a portable ozonator or Aran Jector in the bath helps immensely. One kilogram of Himalayan Fine Granulated Salt on the new moon is claimed to pull out a lot of toxins.

# Salt and Soda Bath

This is what I recommend for a gentle, soothing bath that will reduce inflammation, relax the muscles and clear dead auric energy or accumulated negative thoughts. Draw a bath as hot as is comfortable for you and add to the water while it is filling, 1 cup of Baking Soda and 1 cup of Sea Salt. Both are available inexpensively in bulk. Soak in this tub for 20 minutes or more. For best results take your bath right before bedtime to guarantee a restful night's sleep.

# Water

Hydration is essential for the body to function regularly and most people I see today are woefully under hydrated. In his book "Your Body's Many Cries For Water", Dr. F. Batmanghelidj sites dehydration as the cause of many complaints such as low back pain, inflammation, dyspepsia and rheumatoid arthritis and a gamut of other common ailments. Stress is a major cause of dehydration and often we try to feed the body's thirst with carbonated and caffeinated drinks which will cause more dehydration. These types of beverages, often containing a high sugar content, do not serve the needs of the vascular and lymph systems that have to drive the body's supply of oxygen and glucose energy.

Drinking at least 8 glasses of pure filtered water a day is good sense and we can increase its absorbability if we add good salt for the electrolyte content. The best way to do this is to make up a batch of 'Sole'. Here's how to make a batch that can be used every day.

# Sole Water

- *Take a quart mason jar and layer the bottom ¼ with Himalayan Pink salt crystals. These are available at your local health food store or on line.*

- *Add filtered water to the top of the jar and let it sit on the counter over night. The salt will gradually dissolve over time.*

- *The next day take 1 TBLS of this solution and add it to 1 QT of filtered water. (Use a non metal wooden spoon for this operation)*

- *Drink this diluted saltwater solution through out the day.*

To your daily water you may also add a ¼ tsp of Chia or Flax seeds. These become mucilaginous through out the day and help to breakdown the molecules of the water making it 'soft' and more available to penetrate and hydrate the cells in the body.

Choose a glass bottle. Recent studies have shown that chemicals which have been linked to breast cancer, where found in the breast tissue of women who kept plastic drinking bottles in their cars. The deadly toxins are released when the bottles are repeatedly heated by the sun. Replace your water daily and remember to drink at least 6 to 8 glasses or one quart each day.

# Qigong and Tai Chi Chuan

These marshal arts are the health generating and rejuvenating exercises from the East and are an important part of a program to clear cancer from the body. They are essential for maintaining flexibility and strength as we age. 'Qi' or 'Chi' means energy. In Yoga, it is called 'Prana'. 'Gong' or 'Kung' means work. Therefore, Qigong means the exercise of your internal energy. It is a 5,000-year-old Chinese healthcare modality that has both endured the test of time and is making a tremendous resurgence at the threshold of the 21st Century.

The benefits of Qigong are increasingly recognized for enhancing fitness in mind and body, developing vitality for sports and sex, and helping in the cure of stress as well as degenerative and chronic diseases. Millions practice Qigong in China as a daily morning routine. In many countries it is used successfully to relieve stress and to treat diseases such as diabetes, hypertension and cancer.

I practice and teach Shibashi Qigong, which is based in the philosophy of Tai Chi and extracts some of the best movements from Yang style Tai Chi Chuan. There are 18 moves that are easy to learn and the full program only takes about 20 minutes. It is an extremely important tool for anyone recovering from illness and to maintain vital energy into old age.

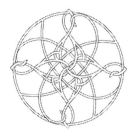

# CHAPTER 18

# AFFIRMATIONS AND VISUALIZATIONS

*"PORTA ITINERI LONGISSIMA EST"*
(The first step being taken, the rest is easy)

Erasmus

## AFFIRMATIONS

I N a previous chapter we have already discussed the power of mind over matter remembering Deepak Chopra's powerful quote,

"Where the mind goes, the body must follow." What we say and do, or what is said and done to us, affects our mind. Then emotions kick in and the body acts like an instant barometer, reacting in subtle, and sometimes not so subtle ways, with physical responses. The good news is that when we become aware of this, we can turn it to our advantage by using positive affirmations and visualizations to stimulate a positive physical response.

There is an old music hall song that I remember hearing many times on the radio as a child growing up in England and it had a profound effect on me. It is about a fellow who sets out from his house one morning feeling well and happy to be alive. "My word, I do feel fine!" he sings joyfully, as he sets off to begin his day. Along the way he is greeted by one friend after another who tells him he looks ill. "My word, you do look queer" they say, "My word, you do look strange."

The songs tempo gets slower and more turgid as he repeats what they have told him and pretty soon he begins to feel sick. "My word, I do feel queer?" he sings, and he starts to turn around to go home. Just then he meets a friend in good spirits who tells him how great he looks. In fact he's never seen him looking better! The song tempo lifts with his spirits and pretty soon he's off down the road again singing happily, "My word, I do feel fine! My word, I do feel fine!"

The power of suggestion is very impressive on our psyche and just as we want to avoid doomsayers, we want to encourage a positive attitude from others and ourselves. It is well known that some patients who are given a prognosis of immanent death in a number of weeks or months, give up on life and, very often, die on the exact date forecast by the doctors.

Affirmations are powerful tools for impressing the mind if they are positive and heartfelt. The sub-conscious mind is always listening to what the conscious mind speaks and tends to believe that what it hears is true. In the beginning you may not feel positive and hopeful but the repeated saying of a positive phrase is the same as the power of prayer or mantra. It will become real the more attention you give to it.

Set aside time every day to repeat uplifting and positive phrases to yourself, inwardly or aloud, and/or read life positive affirmations that have meaning for you. Doing this before quiet time, meditation, or just prior to sleep, can be the most beneficial because it locks into the unconscious and works on a subtle level during the night. It is best, at first, to say the phrase out loud, quietly to yourself, but once you become more proficient, memorizing and repeating the words in your mind over and over will work just as well.

The wonderful books by Louise Hay are full of affirmations for every situation and I highly recommend them. Here's one of my favorites, slightly adapted by me, which I have used every morning, prior to a short meditation time.

> In the infinity of life where I am
> All is perfect, whole and complete.
> I accept health as the natural state of my Being.
> I now consciously release any mental pattern
> which could express as disease in any way.
> I love and approve of myself.
> I love and approve of my body.
> I feed it nourishing foods and beverages
> And I exercise it in ways that are fun.
> I recognize my body as a wondrous, magnificent machine
> And I feel privileged to live in it.
> I love to sleep well at night
> And I love lots of daytime energy.
> All is well in my world.

Be sure to always use the present tense, as if your desires were occurring now. Make up your own affirmations to suit your situation. Here is an exercise you can do called the Sun Wheel. On a blank sheet of paper, draw a circle in the center about 2 inches in diameter. Write the word Sun Wheel in the centre of the circle. Now make up your own affirmations and write them spreading out from the edges of the circle like the rays of the sun. Here are some sample affirmations for you to use. There is also a blank Sun Wheel for your own affirmations at the end of this chapter.

> I give thanks for my healing.
> I now accept perfect health in my body.
> Every day in every way I am stronger and healthier.
> I now make a complete recovery.
> I am on the right path to wellness.
> My body knows how to heal itself.

I listen to my body and do what it tells me.
Others have healed themselves and so can I.
I am a Self-Healing Being who is experiencing improved health each
and every day.

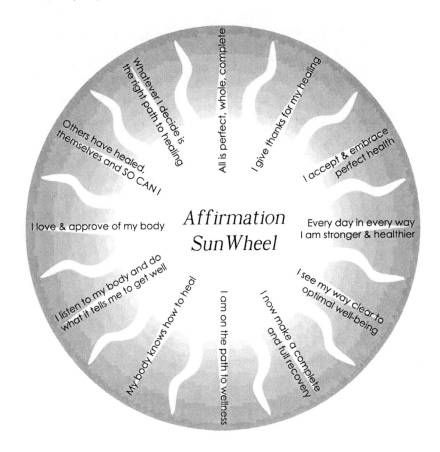

Figure 2: Affirmation Sun Wheel

The affirmations you make up yourself can be the most powerful. Spend some time writing and creating your own Sunwheel and keep it handy to look at every day. Even if you don't believe the affirmation, your body will respond positively. Find the ones that resonate with you and say them randomly throughout the day. They will soon become second nature and begin to reprogram your body.

# VISUALIZATIONS

Images that you can create in your mind's eye can be an even greater healing tool than the spoken word and, done together, they make a formidable combination. Imagine the interior of your body as the miracle that it truly is. There are trillions of cells, each with its own function, operating day in and day out, to keep your body healthy. We don't give much thought to our organs working tirelessly or our heart pumping blood around our body every second, 24/7 for years on end. The bodies' inner workings never take a vacation, so take a moment to give some appreciation to this system that is supporting your life here on Earth.

Maybe you are fighting a disease that is wreaking havoc with the normal functions that previously worked so well? Close your eyes and conjure up an image, like a movie, of the interior of your body with its myriad blood vessels, lymph system channels, plasma and blood cells, flowing effortlessly under your skin. Now create a picture of the precious leukocytes, the defense system known as killer 'T' cells, immediately mobilizing to attack any cancerous invaders. Mobilize these helpers into an army and see them as gleaming, white cells of fire. Now send them to that part of your body that needs help. Imagine them seeking out and destroying any cancer cells that have got out of control. See them eat up the cancer cells like little Pac men and deposit the detritus into the lymph system to be expelled by the eliminative organs. Imagine the part of your body that is sick begin to radiate with energy and light as it cleanses itself and returns to full, vibrant health.

You can do this with the food that you eat or the medicine you take by praying over it before you take it into your body. Then visualize the positive effects that it will have on your health by bringing nutritive power and healing energy where ever it is needed.

During my own healing I made a trip to Vancouver, Canada to attend a special healing seminar. It was given by a young man, still in his teens, who wrote a book about his ability to heal people by visualizing images of light and fire burning up the disease in their bodies. The weekend sessions were packed to capacity and I found myself like many others trying to be early for each session to get as close to the stage as possible. If you were lucky you could be chosen to go up on stage and be screened by his ability to look into the body and see the trouble spots.

His group healing powers were highly touted and each day he would spend some minutes sending healing energy to the audience while we sat quietly visualizing healing in our bodies. I went home having felt nothing palpable from these sessions, but with the understanding that this young man impressed on all of us before we left - that everyone possesses the innate ability to heal others and themselves with the visualization techniques that he taught us. His book is called Dreamhealer and information can be found on the website www.dreamhealer.com .

One of the techniques worked particularly well for me. It was to imagine a bolt of lightning coming from above and entering the crown of your head. From there see it infusing your body with energy and traveling to all parts, but particularly to that area of your body that needs it, destroying any cancer that may be there. See and smell the smoke and burning tissue of the lightning strike as it continues to course through your body repeatedly, unstoppable in its power to destroy cancer cells.

I developed a visualization of my own that I adapted from this. Sit quietly before meditation or simply close your eyes any time you are somewhere quiet. See and feel a bluish-white or green-gold light enter the crown of the head and slowly travel downwards, infusing every cell and tissue with healing energy that burns away any disease and replaces it with vibrant health, Flood the body continuously with this light until it is all the way down to your toes and extends out several inches from the body's surface into the etheric body and beyond. Do this regularly every day whenever you have a quiet moment.

Make up your own visuals for whatever works for you. If you have trouble visualizing images, use your capacity to feel, which will probably be more developed than others. Be creative and go with what feels right. Never underestimate the mind's visualizing power to heal.

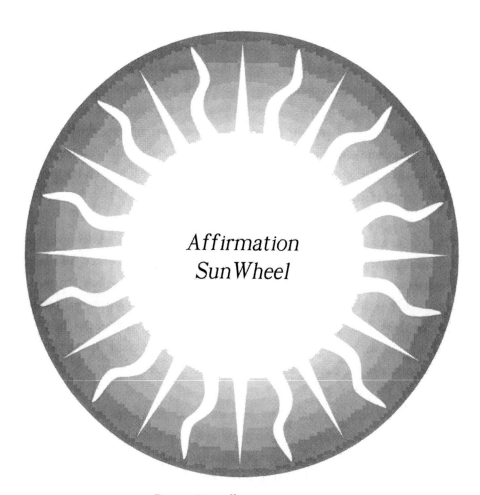

Figure 3: Your Affirmation Sun Wheel

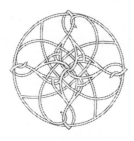

# CHAPTER 19

# SOLAR POWER & SUN GAZING

THE sun has been much maligned of late because of the deterioration of the ozone layer and the heating up of the planet. However, the sun's power to heal has been known for centuries. Hundreds of years ago our ancestors lived out doors year round and learned to value the sun's contribution to plant growth and the health of human beings.

Vitamin D from the sun's rays is absolutely necessary for the body's immune response and recent studies have shown that many people are deficient in this essential vitamin. The best time to take in this vital nutrient is between the hours of 11 am and 3 pm by exposing your torso, and particularly your solar plexus, for a period of up to 15 minutes. Open your palms and imagine the sun pouring energy into the hands and filling up your heart. Breathe deeply and slowly throughout this process, keeping the eyes closed.

The second exercise involves gazing at the sun. I know! I know! Your mom told you never to do this, but sun gazing is an ancient, esoteric healing practice that she didn't know about. It produces changes in the metabolic processes of the body that are key to building vitality and immune strength. If done consistently over time (and this of course depends on the season and the amount of Sun available where you live), it can produce valuable results.

<u>WHEN:</u>…Only choose the times one hour after the sun rises in the morning when you can first view it appearing on the horizon, and one hour before the sun sets in the evening as it sinks in the west. This is when the suns rays are filtered by the earth's stratosphere and the eyes are able to tolerate the light.

<u>CAUTION: Doing this at any other time of the day can damage the cornea of the eyes and I strongly advise against it!</u>

<u>HOW:</u> If possible stand with the feet slightly apart in a relaxed posture and face towards the sun. It can be done sitting if you are too weak, but standing allows the energy to better circulate throughout the whole body. Gaze at the morning sun with your eyes almost closed and slowly open them using the eye lashes as a filter. Begin slowly to open the eyes more until you can gaze at the ball of the sun without filtering. The sun is a reddish orb at this time in the morning and is safe to look at. DO THIS FOR <u>TEN SECONDS</u> ONLY, in small bursts at first until your eyes become accustomed to the energy. Begin adding twenty seconds a day until you can do a total of ten minutes each day.

You can also simultaneously hold your hands open toward the sun to receive the energy through the palms. Stand with your bare feet on the earth to increase the healing power of the earth's magnetic energy.

Continue building your ability to gaze uninterrupted for periods of 10 minutes in the morning and/or evening over a period of 6 months. This time schedule will depend a lot on the weather and your time availability of course, but you will feel the healing energy very early in the process and the rule is to take it easy and increase your capacity to gaze slowly day by day.

The Ancients viewed this practice as a nutritional source of health and longevity feeding the brain and body. If practiced for long periods you will experience healing on all levels. See the website by Hira Ratan Manek www.solarhealing.com He has lived on sun energy alone for many years. The book "<u>The Earth was Flat</u>," by Mason Howe Dwinell L.Ac. is another good resource for learning more about this healing method.

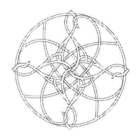

# CHAPTER 20

# THE CANCER CURE PIONEERS

## WILHELM REICH

*"Love, work and knowledge are
the wellsprings of our life.
They should also govern it."*

Wilhelm Reich

## BLOOD, BREATH AND SEX

IN the Europe of the early 1920's, Wilhelm Reich was a medical scientist, biologist, sociologist and leading light in the nascent beginnings of psychoanalysis and an early student of Sigmund Freud, whom he would eventually break from to follow his own theories. He was the "father" of the present day somatic (body oriented) therapies with dozens of spin-offs broadly collected under what is now called Bio-Energetics.

A meticulous researcher and pathologist, his early experiments with cancer patients in America and his discovery of 'orgone' energy, led to a huge breakthrough in cancer cure and treatment in the 1930's and 40's. His subsequent vilification by the American Medical Association and the defamation of his work, even to this day, is a travesty of justice and a sad statement about the suppression of information in the field of cancer research over the last hundred years.

In his ground-breaking book 'The Cancer Biopathy', Reich postulates his theory of the biophysical, psychic and sexual connotations behind all disease and particularly cancer. Fastidious and scrupulously honest about his failures as well as his successes, he documented case histories of patients he treated, with instruments and equipment he designed himself at his Institute for Orgone Research in Virginia.

His discovery and scientific documentation of 'orgone energy', known for centuries in Eastern philosophy and medical practice as 'prana' or Qi ( pronounced 'chi'), the vital life force that pervades the Universe, and his subsequent experiments using it to heal cancer patients, was the early discovery and recognition of the mind/body connection, or 'quantum' theory of healing.

Reich studied the blood of cancer patients through a high powered micro-scope and discovered a common microbe he called T-bacilli, that attacked and destroyed healthy cells. He learned that healthy red blood cells that were infused with 'bion', derived from orgone energy, were lacking in cancerous or precancerous bodies and would attack the T-bacilli. The unhealthy blood cells, what we might term today as the immune response system, could be rejuvenated in a sick person by flooding the body with a concentration of this natural orgone energy found in the atmosphere.

The newly infused red blood cells then exhibited a characteristic blue hemi-sphere and went to work destroying the T-bacilli in the cancer patient. Riech developed the 'Orgone Accumulator' for this purpose, a large cabinet constructed of layers of conductive materials in its walls. A person could sit in this enclosed cabinet and receive concentrated amounts of the 'orgone' energy pulled in from the atmosphere, thus rejuvenating the blood of the patient.

The treatments were meticulously documented along with subsequent blood analysis and were always given free of charge. With these daily treatments Reich documented many successful cancer cures and dramatic reversals of tumor growth. The health of the blood system was always an important factor in a patient's recovery, but so also was the patient's emotional attitude. When a patient was able to combine a conscious awareness of their psychological structure in a positive healing environment, they invariably got well.

When fear, anxiety and psychic neurosis were permitted to dominate the person's life, successful treatment was not possible or seriously delayed. Along with this positive attitude toward healing, Reich stressed the importance of the breath in oxygenating the blood and rejuvenating the cells and, more importantly, in releasing stored up emotional trauma locked in the muscular tissue of the body.

He was one of the first to recognize this mind/body connection and developed early therapies using breath work to break down this unconscious 'character armoring' that prevented the patient from fully experiencing life. These therapies included deep diaphragmatic breathing and vocal expression to release emotions trapped in the body by years of emotional and sexual repression.

A common thread in cancer patients was what Reich called 'sexual stasis.' This was the absence of healthy sexual release or the inability to experience full body orgasm. He postulated that this lack of true sexual pleasure and loving gratification in people's lives led to psychic stress and physical disease. These theories were a statement of the sociological and political state of the times, the suppression of happiness and joy by an authoritarian, sex suppressive, common society. They are as present in the world today as they were in Reich's time.

Reich's life and work, briefly described here, are worth further reading and can be accessed at www.wilhelmreichmuseum.com . Whether you believe in his theories or not, it is worth noting that 70 years ago Reich was way ahead of his time. He was an early pioneer of the modern day theories about the importance of blood pathology and the commonality of the oxygen deficient, anaerobic human body in the current cancer epidemic.

My own experience with Reichian Breathwork and the study of Reich's work, leads me to express my deep appreciation and gratitude for his genius. I feel that my emotional and physical health improved in large part to an understanding of the vital role played by 'blood, breath and sex' in the healing of the human body.

To make use of 'orgone' in the healing of any disease get an Orgone Blanket or Orgone Accumulator that will intensify the free orgone energy and transfuse the body with its healing power. These are available in California and links to this equipment and more information about Reich and the latest technology available can be found at www.orgonics.com and www.orgonomicscience.org

# DR. MAX GERSON

*"I see in Dr. Max Gerson one of the most*
*eminent geniuses in the history of medicine"*
Dr. Albert Schweitzer

Max Gerson was born in Germany in 1881 and he died in the US in 1959. He came to this country in the 1940's and was originally treating people for tuberculosis with a special diet he had used successfully to treat his own migraine headaches. He started treating cancer patients on the insistence of a cancer client who thought it would work for her, and it did. He began to take in other cancer patients and treated them with a soup that was originally used by Hippocrates and also introduced fresh vegetable juices and raw foods.

Over the years he successfully treated hundreds of cancer victims, many in the advanced stages after western therapy had failed them. The Gerson Institute operates in Tijuana, Mexico and is run to this day by his surviving daughter,

Charlotte, an amazing woman now in her 80's who is tireless and determined in her advancement of his principles.

Gerson therapy is one of the original *metabolic* therapies, using a special diet, supplements, and the coffee enema, to cure terminal cases of cancer. Ninety percent of his cancer cases were far advanced (terminal), and overall his cure rate was about 50%, which is exceptional because he counted all of his patients, not just those who lived for a year or more. This percentage is far higher than current day orthodox treatments and higher than most alternative cancer treatments!!

In his own words…..*"The ideal task of cancer therapy is to restore the function of the oxidizing systems in the entire organism. This, of course, is difficult to accomplish. It involves the following: 1) detoxification of the whole body, 2) providing the essential mineral contents of the potassium group, 3) adding oxidizing enzymes continuously as long as they are not reactivated and built in the body (in the form of green leaf juice and fresh calf's liver juice). This will create a near normal condition of the oxidizing system in the body, to which malignant cells with the fermentation system cannot adapt."*

*Dr. Max Gerson, A Cancer Therapy, 5th Edition, page 7*

You can read more about this program and successful cases in "A Cancer Therapy – Results of Fifty Cases" by Max Gerson and "The Gerson Therapy" by Charlotte Gerson and Morton Walker D.M.P or go to www.gerson.org for more information.

# ROYAL RIFE

*"Having spent every dime I earned in my research*
*for the benefit of mankind, I have ended up a pauper -*
*but I achieved the impossible and I would do it again.*

Royal Raymond Rife, 1967

In the 1930's Dr. Royal Rife, a microbiologist, built an electron microscope of enormous power that could magnify images up to 4,000X. This was twice the power of microscopes available at that time and still more powerful than the most sophisticated instruments built today. With it he was able to discover that an aberrant microbe infiltrated certain cells causing them to become deviant and, by denying the bodies normal messages, start to form cancerous tumors.

He then developed a machine that created very high radio frequency sounds. When these frequencies were passed though the cellular system, they caused the aberrant cancer sells to vibrate and destroy the microbe inside it, thereby returning it to a normal healthy cell. His initial studies were done on rats but he eventually started to apply these radio frequencies to cancer patients because they were completely safe and, except for the die off effect of the dead material leaving the body, caused no side effects. His first 16 patients were all cured by this method; an incredible 100% record.

This is when his notoriety came to the attention of the AMA and the FDA. After he refused to cooperate with the authorities to sell his ideas to them, one of his clinics was mysteriously burned to the ground. Equipment and records were routinely stolen and he was threatened with legal proceedings. Finally he was prosecuted in court for practicing medicine without a license and his equipment and files were destroyed along with the threatened persecution of other doctors who were following his protocols.

This is another sad tale of big medical business interests afraid that simple cures would interfere with their money making endeavors. You can find plenty of information about this crime on the internet. Rife himself was hounded into obscurity and exiled himself in New Mexico for the remainder of his life. He died in 1971.

During his time Rife was insistent on securing the right frequencies for each disease and this is still the most important rule today for targeting the cancer cells. The latest equipment comes with manuals detailing the frequencies for each disease but this is still a random affair. I still use the Rife Machine BX 200/400 today and experiment with various frequencies by muscle testing. It cost me $2500 in 2005.

The latest equipment I have found in my research is the GB 4000, 20 MHz Sweep/Function Generator available from The Frequency Store at 1-800 477 0066. It is also about $2500 but you get a lot more for your money with this latest technology.

For specific protocols of how to use this equipment I recommend the wonderful website www.cancertutor.com put out by the Independent Cancer Research Foundation run by R. Webster Kehr, one of the pre-eminent cancer researchers today. His website is undoubtedly one of the best places for information about alternative protocols for cancer.

# DR. WILLIAM DONALD KELLEY, DDS

*"If we don't change the whole course of health care,
we won't have accomplished a thing"*

Dr. William Kelley

Dr. Kelley first came to prominence in the 60's with the publication of his book "One Answer to Cancer", which he wrote after curing himself of pancreatic and liver cancer. His theories of cancer healing are based on what he learned from Gerson's therapy and has become known today as Metabolic Medicine. This is the science of understanding a person's metabolic type and how they digest certain foods for nutrition and protein absorption. He stipulates that there are ten types. Once you begin to follow his prescribed diet for your type and take the pancreatic enzymes he developed, along with cleansing the colon with coffee enemas, you can begin to regain health.

Depending on what stage your cancer is at you will take a lot of supplements, up to 100 per day and the cost is not cheap. However, the quality has been rigorously tested and they are the best. Do not try to doctor yourself and change the program because you think your way is better. Success rates are high because the patients are disciplined and stick with the program.

He worked at this for over 40 years until his death through suspicious circumstance in 2007 and has over 30,000 successful cures. He was attacked and persecuted constantly by the medical establishment for his ideas but his record speaks for itself. His program is called "Metabolic Medicines Cancer Cure Program" and you must follow it exactly for best results. His revised book "Cancer : Curing the Incurable" and the program supplements are available online at www.newcenturypromotions.com or from New Century Promotions Inc., 3711 Alta Loma Dr., Bonita, Ca 91902 Tel. 1 800 768 8484

# THE MODERN PIONEERS

## MAJID ALI, M.D.

As I was preparing this book for printing and, as usual, by a seemingly chance association with a person I was care-giving for, I came across her collection of books by Dr Majid Ali. For several weeks I didn't take any notice of them until one afternoon as I was preparing some food for her, I took one of his books off the kitchen shelf and browsed through it. What I read immediately struck a cord with me and I became very excited as I began to question my friend about Dr Ali and his theories on health, aging and cancer.

Unquestionably Dr. Ali is one of the most experienced and brilliant practitioners of Integrative Medicine in America today. He is the Director of the Institute of Integrative Medicine in New York, Denville and New Jersey. He has over 50 years of work in the established medical field as a physician, pathologist and surgeon and his work and study with cancer patients put him, in my mind, as the authoritative leader in cancer research, integrative medicine and preventative care.

In a practice that he terms molecular or metabolic medicine he incorporates nutrition, environmental medicine, limbic exercise, autonomic regulation and breathing, oxygen therapy and spiritual contemplation along with his first hand knowledge of surgery, chemotherapy and radiation when these might be deemed necessary. There is no substitute for experience and knowledge and Majid Ali has these qualities more than any medical practitioner I have researched.

My publishing was delayed as I immersed myself in his books and particularly his Tetralogy of Cancer called "The Crab, Oxygen and Cancer" Volume 1 and 2. In it he lays out his theories for the major causes for the disease called cancer and how it can be treated. He is scathingly honest about the sometimes deceptive cancer practices of the established oncology hospitals as well as alternative, natural health practitioners who give false and misleading claims in the treatment of cancer.

His basic theory focuses on the bio-terrain of the body and how cancer cells are generated by environmental pollutants, synthetic ingredients in our food, the air we breathe and even the negative thoughts we have. He states that the three major destroyers of normal cells are;

1 Acidosis; too much acidity

2 Oxidosis; too many free radicals ( environmental toxins)

3 Dysoxygenosis; malfunction of cells due to lack of oxygen.

His oxystatic therapeutics in his clinics seek to restore oxygen homeostasis with hydrogen peroxide/vitamin/mineral and ozone intravenous and intramuscular injections, as well as EDTA chelation therapy to remove heavy metals from the body. He emphasizes liver and bowel detoxification and individualized nutritional and nutrient support.

His books are easy to read and he uses wonderful metaphors, titles and anecdotes that both excite and illuminate. It would be impossible for me to do him justice in this short overview and so as I humbly bow to his enormous contribution to Integrative Medicine I urge you to visit his website . www. majidali.com, and read his extensive treatises on cancer, aging and health, especially the book "The Crab, Oxygen and Cancer, Vol. 2: *The Oxygen Protocol for the Treatment of Cancer*".

Many of his theories for treatment parallel my own experience in my recovery and go way beyond them. For anyone with cancer or researching cancer therapies, his books are required reading

# ANDREAS MORITZ

Andreas Moritz is a medical intuitive and practitioner of Ayurveda, Iridology, Shiatsu, and Vibrational Medicine and perhaps the most remarkable healer and teacher to appear on the alternative health scene in the last five years. I found him originally through his book "The Amazing Gallbladder and Liver Flush" whose protocols I tell you about in the chapter on cleansing the body.

The next book I read, "Cancer is NOT a Disease – It is a Defense Mechanism", plunged me deep into the '*New Medicine*' principles of mind/body medicine and the power of faith and belief in healing the body. This book posits that the cancer symptoms that form tumors in the body are really an attempt to deal with congestion and toxins and are actually trying a last ditch effort to save the body from death.

Besides being an expose of conventional 'treatments' which harm the body, it gives directions in how to heal and how to cleanse. It points out the roles of fear, frustration, low self-worth and repressed anger in the origination of cancer and most importantly the spiritual lessons behind cancer. Even beyond this it delves briefly into the understanding of a radical spiritual viewpoint to take us beyond the emotional and egoic blocks that suppress our true nature. In his book "Lifting the Veil of Duality", he goes further into an exploration of the role of duality in our daily lives and opens up the whole question of how we live in separation from ourselves and others. This book is true healing to the soul and will take you closer to the real meaning of life and health.

His other books and talks, including the comprehensive "Timeless Secrets of Health and Rejuvenation", are all invaluable reading for anyone suffering from disease. He is an accomplished artist and his paintings are created to heal. Check out more at www.ener-chi.com

# DR. NICHOLAS GONZALEZ

Dr. Nicholas J Gonzalez M.D was a second year medical student when he met William Donald Kelley, an eccentric dentist who had cured himself of pancreatic cancer. In the 1960's and 70's Dr. Kelley developed an intensive program for treating cancer using pancreatic enzymes and nutritional approaches. These protocols are further elaborated upon in the following chapter on Metabolic Medicine.

Dr. Gonzalez then spent 5 years researching into thousands of records of Dr. Kelley's patients. What he found convinced him of the successful potential of Kelley's program. He also discovered that the original progenitor of enzyme therapy was Dr. John Beard, a Scottish embryologist. In 1911 Beard said that trypsin, a proteolytic enzyme, was the body's main defense against cancer and he produced a number of papers laying out his theories. Unfortunately he was ahead of his time and his ideas were rejected by the mainstream establishment.

After studying Dr. Beard's literature and working closely with Dr. Kelley, and seeing him reverse cancer, Dr. Gonzalez walked away from conventional medicine and made a commitment to go into alternative cancer research using the enzyme theories. His book, "One Man Alone : An Investigation of Nutrition, Cancer and William Donald Kelley", is available from New Spring Press. Dr. Gonzalez is a brave innovator and has practiced in New York since 1987. His website is www.Dr-gonzalez.com

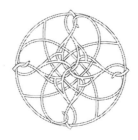

# CHAPTER 21

# METABOLIC MEDICINE

*"Nothing cures cancer—only your body.*
*My program and products are designed to help restore*
*the body to a healthy position so the body can*
*overcome the cancer. People, however, prostitute*
*the program, play doctor, make changes and then*
*wonder why my program did not work"*

Dr. William Donald Kelley

IN the previous chapter on the Cancer Cure Pioneers I told you a little bit about the history of Metabolic Medicine and its founder Dr. William Kelley. Now I will tell you why I think it is the 'go to' remedy for any cancer, regardless of its stage and why I recommend it as an integral part of The Natural Cancer Recovery Program. Often patients have tried conventional allopathic methods of chemotherapy and radiation without success and many of them have also tried to supplement other natural alternative methods to no avail. At this late stage, serious intervention is required to turn the disease around. This is often when I suggest incorporating Dr. Kelley's protocol.

However, when drugs or conventional treatments have been used, the body's natural defenses have been seriously compromised and it is a much more difficult task to turn the health around. Better to begin this program as soon as cancer is detected.

Although I did not use it as part of my own initial recovery, as recently as the spring of 2010 my routine HCG Urine test came back positive. It was only slightly over the base line for cancer cells present in the body and although I was following many of the protocols I recommend in this book and felt very healthy, I implemented the Metabolic Program to test its efficacy for myself. Now I could work with cancer patients on a deeper and more knowledgeable level.

The result was a boost in energy and, along with a special diet and the kidney and liver flushes, a new and vibrant feeling of health. Friends began to ask me what I was doing to look so good. I stayed on the program for 4 months, doing the coffee enemas every day. The positive response to the program also gave me a sense of empowerment and self control that I always tell cancer patients they will feel when they begin to take charge of their own health in this way.

Now a little about the program specifics. The basic foundation of Dr Kelly's program are the enzymes. There are two types of enzymes, PEP and Solzyme. They are identical except that the PEP contains glandular while the Solzyme does not. If you have any of the hormone driven cancers i.e. breast, prostate, cervical or ovarian, you should take the Solzyme which does not contain the glandular formula. Taking the PEP with the glandular formula runs the risk of feeding the afore mentioned cancers because of their hormonal origin. The PEP can be used with many of the other cancers.

Dr. Kelley stressed that there are 4 things that are set in stone to do the program correctly and these must be done everyday without fail until the cancer is overcome. These are:

1. Beta-1, 3-D Glucan capsules first thing upon arising in the morning. (100 lbs 2 caps, 150 lbs 3 caps, 200 lbs plus 4/5 caps)

2. Formula Solozyme Pancreatic Enzymes one hour before breakfast, 6 to 8 in Stages 1 and 2; 10 to 12 enzymes in Stages 3 and 4.

The enzymes are taken upon arising, before the morning enema. Between a half hour and an hour before each meal, between each meal, and again before bed. A total of seven times each day.

3. Phosphoric Acid (Phosflow) and Protein drink, 1 dropperful in the drink.

4. Coffee enema in the morning.

Here is a simplified explanation of why you do these 4 steps in this order.

First, the Beta Glucan acts as an immune booster and prepares the body to efficiently accept the enzyme process. (Contraindications include pregnant women and any persons having received an organ transplant.)

Second, the special formula enzymes developed by Dr. Kelley have a pancreatic enzyme called Chymotrypsin which breaks down the protective protein shield the cancer cells have formed around themselves and makes them vulnerable to attack by the NK (natural killer) cells previously enhanced by the Beta Glucan.

Now the Phosphoric Acid added to the highly potent protein drink dilates the blood vessels to help transport the dead cancer cells to the eliminative organs of the liver, kidneys, lymph, and large and small intestines.

Finally the coffee enema stimulates the bile production of the liver and gallbladder and they simultaneously eliminate the toxins by flushing them into the colon and out through elimination.

<u>You may feel worse before you feel better!</u>

You are systematically breaking down the cancer cells and excess toxic debris in the body and it has to leave the body somehow. It is eliminated via the enemas, urine, sweat, nails and hair. When it is circulating in the blood and lymph you may feel 'die off' in the form of nausea, aches and pains, headaches, dizziness, irritability. This is a *good* thing. It means the program is working. If you feel too toxic you must stop taking the enzymes for 5 days. Let the body catch up and release its toxic build up. Drink plenty of water and do enemas, sweats, salt scrubs and get plenty of rest.

Then begin the program of taking the enzymes again for a period of 21 days and then rest for 5. You must do this for a minimum of 6 months to a year. And even then, depending on your situation, you must continue with a modified program of enzyme and diet. Recovery from cancer can take 2 to 4 yrs and even then you must be *vigilant* for the rest of your life.

There is also a specific diet which closely follows the diet of The Natural Cancer Recovery Program detailed in other chapters. Kelley's theory of Metabolic Typing matches the Ayurvedic principles of individual body types and personalities. Diets are selected for each body type based on a sympathetic or para-sympathetic body type.

Metabolic Medicine recommends no red or white meat for the first 6 months but fresh wild caught fish is acceptable 2 or 3 times a week.

No dairy. Replace this with Almond or Rice milk but watch out for the sweetener Raw Cane Juice even if it says organic. A better choice is rice syrup that can be found in some Rice drinks. If you have breast, prostate, ovarian or cervical cancer—no eggs since these contain hormones. Eggs are acceptable in all other cancers.

No fruit except berries. All berries are acceptable since these are high in antioxidants. No russet or white potatoes since these turn to sugar very quickly. Substitute yams and sweet potatoes. Eat all the vegetables you can but eliminate corn. Bread should be sprouted and nut butters are OK except Peanut Butter which is a legume and difficult to digest. As many vegetable juices as you can handle, but no fruit juice. Nutritional supplements should be taken and tailored to the individual's specific needs.

This is a brief outline of Metabolic Medicine and one can order the program materials and use it in conjunction with the daily Cancer Recovery Program outlined in this book. One source of help is the inimitable Charles Attal at New Century Promotions where you can order the enzymes. Charles is a cancer survivor in his 80's. He is a true gentleman and a wise and tireless source of information for the cancer patient. Give him a call at 619-479-7852 or 1-800-768-8484 or email at www.charlesattal@cox.net .As always he will be happy to answer any questions you may have. The website is www.newcenturypromotions.com

Dr Kelley's book is *"Cancer: Curing the Incurable"*. THIS IS YOUR BIBLE. READ AND RE-READ THIS BOOK FOR A DETAILED DESCRIPTION OF HOW TO DO THIS PART OF THE CANCER RECOVERY PROGRAM!

# PART III

---

# THE PROGRAM

## WHAT YOU CAN
## DO NOW
## IF YOU HAVE CANCER!

*If you panic, you probably won't make it.*

Majid Ali, M.D.

# ATTITUDE

"The longer I live, the more I realize the impact of attitude on life. Attitude, to me, is more important than facts. It is more important than the past, than education, than money, than circumstances, than failures, than successes, than what other people say or do. It is more important than appearance, giftedness or skill. It will make or break a company, church or home. The remarkable thing is we have a choice every day regarding the attitude we will embrace for that day. We cannot change our past; we cannot change the fact that people will act a certain way. We cannot change the inevitable. The only thing we can do is play on the one string we have, and that is our attitude. I am convinced that life is 10% what happens to me and 90% how I react to it. And so it is with you; we are in charge of our attitude."
We are in charge of our attitude.

Charles Swindoll

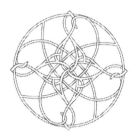

# CHAPTER 22

# TESTING FOR CANCER

## NAVARRO BETA-HCG URINE CANCER TEST

THIS is a safe, cost effective, non-invasive, accurate screening test for cancer. You can do all the western diagnostic tests such as CT/PET scans and MRI's and these may tell the doctors where the tumor is located but they will dose you with the equivalent of 25 X-rays and they will not give you an accurate 'marker' to find out if the alternative regimen you are using is working satisfactorily.

HCG stands for Human Chorionic Gonadotrophin. This test was developed by Dr. Howard Beard, a bio-chemist and cancer patient. He found that high levels of HCG in the body was a factor in pregnancy, keeping the T-lymphocyte cells from rejecting the fetus. When the baby was due the HCG levels drop dramatically allowing the body to 'reject' the fetus in the birthing process.

Similarly when cancer cells are present in the body in higher than normal numbers, the HCG levels will be high because they are restricting the anti-cancer cell activity of the body's natural defense mechanism. If the level is tested from 0 to 49, the body is working at capacity and the cancer cells are being kept under control. If the marker is above 50 then there is an abnormal amount of cancer cells in the body.

Remember everyone has cancer in their body but it is kept under control by the daily activity of the Natural Killer Cells and T-lymphocytes. The high level of HCG indicates that this activity has been restricted and the cancer cells are proliferating. If you have been diagnosed with cancer, get this test done immediately and then check the level every 7/8 weeks to see if you are making progress. This is a simple way for you to evaluate for yourself the effectiveness of your program. Here is the protocol to follow ;

PROCEDURE: Send urine samples by mail to Dr. Efren F. Navarro for the Beta HCG Urine Immunoassay for Cancer Detection.

1. The specimen should be the first urine after midnight. For women there should be no sexual contact for 12 days before collecting the urine sample. DO NOT SEND A URINE SAMPLE IF THE WOMAN IS PREGNANT. For men, no sexual contact for 18-24 hours before.

2. Mix 50cc (1.75 oz.) of urine with 200cc (7 oz.) of acetone (can be purchased from hardware store or pharmacy) and 5cc (1 teaspoon) of isopropyl Alcohol or 95% ethyl alcohol. Stir and mix well.

3. Let the mixture stand for 2 to 4 hours in the refrigerator until sediment forms in the bottom of the container.

4. Throw off about half of the urine –acetone mixture without losing any of the sediment. Filter the remaining mixture through a coffee filter or a laboratory filter paper to retain the sediment.

5. After filtration, air dry the filter paper with the sediment.

6. Fold the filter and place in a plastic bag

7. If results are wanted quickly, send the specimen by courier (FedEx, UPS, or DHL) or by USPS Global Priority Mail to Dr Navarro together with the patients name age, sex, brief medical history and/

or diagnosis, and a Xerox copy of a money order, cashiers check or check for $50 made out to Erlinda N. Suarez. Otherwise send the specimen by regular Priority Air Mail and allow 4-6 weeks for the test result delivery. (By including your email address you will vastly speed up the result delivery process). Dr Navarro's address is:
Dr. Efren Navarro M.D.
3553 Sinning Street
Morningside Terrace
Santa Mesa, Manila 1016
Philippines
Tel. # 011 632-714-7442 (9pm Eastern – 9am Manila)
Email: efnavmed@gmail.com

8. Mail the money order or check (personal checks drawn on a US bank are accepted) for $50 to

Ms. Erlinda N Suarez
631 Peregrine Dr.
Palatine, IL. 60067-7005

9. The specimen will be tested immediately upon arrival. Results will be sent by email as soon as they become available to the patient's and or physicians email address if they have email addresses. The official report will be sent back by air mail.

The message you get back will say something like "+4 [54.3 I.U.] This number indicates ............etc" The +4 actually means plus or minus 4. According to Bill Henderson's excellent 'Cancer Free' book this is an indication of the labs opinion of the accuracy of the number but he says in his experience the number is much more accurate than that. Once your number is 49 or below you are 'Home Free!'

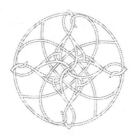

# CHAPTER 23

# COMPLEMENTING CHEMO

I could write a whole chapter on the bludgeoning cancer industry, its profit motives and the unscrupulous funding by the large cancer institutes, but that's not what this book is about. There is also plenty of evidence out there about the negative side effects of chemotherapy, radiation and surgery and the efficacy of this kind of symptom oriented therapy. (See Ralph Moss, Questioning Chemotherapy.)

When it comes right down to it, most cancer sufferers will choose western medicines limited options because that's all they know. That is what the insurance industry supports and that is what people in this country have been led to believe will cure them and some times it does. After all, that's exactly what I did when first diagnosed. However, I would not choose that option again, knowing what I know now.

It takes a great deal of courage to trust in a natural cure and only a small percentage of cancer patients in this country choose that option alone. Many will integrate natural methods to support their treatment and more and more, these days, you will hear the phrase Complementary Alternative Medicine (CAM) being used by the large traditional institutions to describe some of their treatments, and that's a good thing.

'The Natural Cancer Recovery Program' however, is not conducive to chemotherapy and radiation therapy. It would be like a 'tug of war', with one side trying to repair and rebuild the immune system and bring the bio-terrain back into balance and the other side trying to tear it down by adding poison to the body in the hope that the disease will succumb before the person dies from the treatment. I have found it is better to wait until western medicine has run its course, for better or worse, and *then* implement a program to bring the body back to health.

Unfortunately, because western medicine is supported by the insurance industry, and drug treatment in the US is so heavily advertised, many patients choose this first option and only come to alternative medicine after all conventional treatments have failed.

The good news is that there are a number of natural treatments that can be used in conjunction with chemotherapy and radiation, to ameliorate their side effects and actually enhance their effectiveness. Many Oncologists will tell you otherwise. In their opinion the therapies should stand alone and other co-treatments will decrease effectiveness. There have been many studies done that actually support the use of complementary treatments during chemotherapy. Here are some of the things I recommend. You can do further research on them to decide if you want to use them.

- Ginger tea is a great pain reliever and will soothe the nausea caused by chemo and radiation. Peppermint and chamomile also help a queasy stomach.
- Miso Soup with seaweed should be taken every day along with radiation treatments.
- Fresh green juices daily.
- Vitamins C, E and B Complex.
- Fish Oils
- Selenium

- Multi Enzymes (see "The Enzyme Cure" by Lita Lee)
- Vitamin C and K combination. Large dose intra-venous injections with mineral enhancement.
- Infra-red Saunas
- Sound Wave Hypothermia Treatments (Mexico)
- Sono-photo Dynamic Therapy (Hope4cancer, Baja Mexico)
- Liquid Laetrile (Mexico) or crushed apricot seeds for home use.
- Frankincense. Aromatherapy, as a body oil and chewing it orally.

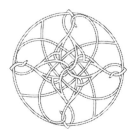

# CHAPTER 24

# FOLLOWING THE DAILY PROGRAM

*We each consist of a metropolis of 50 Trillion citizens, the cells in our body, which could each be considered sentient beings in their own right, yet they act as a community.*"
Bruce Lipton, '<u>Spontaneous Evolution</u>'

I have survived cancer and owe my health to Ayurveda and the many remedies you will find in this book. Subsequently, after 4 more years of research and knowing what I know now I would not hesitate to begin with the ideas you will find in Bill Henderson's wonderful book "<u>Cancer Free</u>".

I highly recommend it as a great resource for information on natural remedies to heal cancer. Easy to read with compelling anecdotes and scientific information, Bill's book is a must read for anyone wanting to know more about natural and inexpensive, self administered cancer therapies. You can go to his website at www.Beating-Cancer-Gently.com and find out more about this tireless cancer crusader and his weekly internet radio show.

I don't agree with everything Bill says because of my own experience in India with Ayurvedic therapies but after discovering his book I use a lot of his suggestions for my own health maintenance. Everyone is unique with respect to their own healing so you must find your own way, but here's what I would do if I were you.

Work with an Ayurvedic or Natural Health Practitioner along side your primary care physician if you have one. Very few medical mainstream doctors or oncologists will support you going your own way so if you are receiving traditional western treatments such as chemotherapy, surgery or radiation, you may have to take a stand and use these alternative methods as integrative, adjunct methods to support your healing.

IMPORTANT *Remember to start the daily program slowly. Start with small doses of the enzymes and monitor your reactions. If you experience anything more extreme than normal toxic cleansing such as headaches, irritableness or nausea, then back off the dose for a few days. Then begin to build up again as your body becomes used to the program.*

Begin by doing 21 consecutive days and then take a 5 day break from the enzymes and enemas. Continue your dietary regime and maintain your sleep and exercise program. Listen to your body. If you feel fatigued, rest. This is normal. You are beginning to build a new body and it takes time.

I offer private consultations and cancer coaching to help you start your program and follow up sessions to support you staying on track. You can also email any questions for me at www.ravenayurveda@gmail.com

# The Daily Program

- 6 -7am. Wake up
- Drink 2-3 glasses of room temperature filtered water
- 3/4 caps of Beta-1, 3-D Glucan
- Meditation and breathing – 20 to 40 minutes

- 6 to 10 Pancreatic Enzymes
- Bathroom – Elimination, scrape tongue and oil massage of the whole body
- 2 tsp Turmeric Powder or Green Barley Powder with one dropper of Phos-flow
- Coffee enema
- Hot and cold shower or warm bath. Brush teeth etc.
- Dry brush skin massage
- Exercise – Rebounder/Qi Gong/Yoga/Walk/Jog
- 6 to 10 Pancreatic Enzymes
- 8 – 8:30 am. Protein Shake or breakfast meal.
- Vitamins and Nutritional Supplements
- Mid-morning vegetable juice or cottage cheese with flax oil and 6 to 10 Pancreatic Enzymes
- Pre-lunch Pancreatic Enzymes
- 12 – 2pm. Fresh cooked lunch with protein
- Mid-afternoon vegetable juice with Pancreatic Enzymes
- Pre-dinner Pancreatic Enzymes
- 6 -7pm. Light evening meal with digestive enzymes
- Relaxation/reading/music/entertainment
- Before bed supplements and Pancreatic Enzymes
- 9:30 – 10pm. Lights out, bedtime

# Ongoing

- Liver flush every 4 weeks on the new moon
- 21 Day Kidney flush every 8 to 10 weeks
- Weekly massage/bodywork/lymph drainage

- Weekly salt scrubs, baths and other cleanses
- Daily exercise, walking, jogging, playing etc.
- Emotional Release Work with a Professional Therapist every week.
- Annual Pancha Karma treatment (*detailed in Chapter 39*)
- Regular reading of Kelly's Cancer-Curing the Incurable.
- *Reminder : Start slowly, build up gradually.*

IMPORTANT : Please start slowly with 3 or 4 enzymes each time. If you feel any reactions like nausea, irritableness or headache, this is normal. Back off the dosage a little and build up slowly again until you can tolerate the full dosage. After 21 days take a break from the enzymes and enemas for 5 days and then begin the cycle again.

# How much will this cost?

The approximate cost of the enzymes will vary depending on the supplier you choose. They will cost between $600 per month for the Pancreas Natural Glandular from ARG and $1200 to $1500 per month for the original Kelly formula called Solzyme which is recommended for the hormonal cancers. Naturally, if you can afford it, go with Kelly's product but the ARG formula worked well for me. The additional supplements and the essential ingredients of your diet will depend on your budget.

# The Essential Ingredients

## Pancreatic Enzymes

These are the foundation of the Metabolic Cure by Dr. William Kelley detailed in Chapter 21. I believe that they are essential in helping the body assimilate and digest the proper plant proteins and minerals when the body is stressed with cancer. Taken as a supplement on an empty stomach they enter the blood stream and digest toxins, stripping the cancer cells of their protective protein coating, enabling the immune system to direct the residue to the kidneys, urinary tract, colon and skin for elimination.

Pancreatic enzymes specifically support the pancreas in its ability to digest cancer cells. They are anti-inflammatory and detoxifying agents that help maintain the healthy pH of the body. You may feel worse in the beginning as the body begins to break down tumor masses, therefore it is essential to seek the help of a health professional who can guide your enzyme supplementation program or buy and read for yourself Dr. Kelly's book 'Cancer; Curing the Incurable'. These enzymes are not cheap but relatively speaking they are a fraction of the cost of conventional treatment and priceless in their ability to help you recover from cancer. Dr. Kelly's original pancreatic formula is distributed exclusively through New Century Promotions and participating health care practitioners. There address is 3711 Alta Loma Drive, Bonita, CA 91902. 800-768-8484 or 619-479-7852. Fax 619-479-3829.

I have found a less expensive formula which I believe works just as well for non-hormonal cancer and is 1/3 the price of Kelly's formula. This same formula is used by Dr Gonzalez's clinic in New York. It is available with a Patient Participation Program through health care practitioners like myself. Ask your health care provider to become a distributer. Call Allergy Research Group, 2300 North Loop Rd. Alameda CA 94502. 800-545-9960 or 510-263-2000 Fax 510-263-2100 www.nutricology.com

# Beta-1, 3-D Glucan

You have to give your body a fighting chance to heal itself and the best way to do that is to build the immune system especially if it has been compromised by chemotherapy and radiation. If you haven't gone that route then you're ahead of the game.

Beta Glucan is derived from a yeast extract in a unique way by Transfer Point Labs. It is the top immune modulator available. Beta Glucan binds to a receptor on the neutrophil immune cells that make up 50/60% of the system. They can recognize cancer cells as fungus and kill them. Natural Killer (NK) cells, macrophages and eosinophils also have these glucan receptor sites, which adds to their effectiveness. You can purchase Beta-1,3-D Glucan in capsules and find out more information by visiting the website www.BetterWayHealth.com

## The Budwig Diet

Flax seed oil and cottage cheese are so easy to obtain you should go out and buy them right now. Make it a habit to eat this powerful combination every day while you are recovering from cancer and use the maintenance amount thereafter.

Use 2/3 cup low fat or 2% fat organic cottage cheese and mix in 6 table-spoons ( 1/3 cup) of fresh refrigerated flax oil. Barleans is the best, but any organic brand will do as long as you find it in the refrigerated section of the store. Keep it refrigerated at home and shake it well each time you use it. Eat it soon after you have blended it and add fruit to taste if you wish. Blueberries are great It can be split into two servings morning and afternoon. Just make it fresh each time. Check out www.BudwigVideos.com or for complete infor-mation go to www.healingcancernaturally.com

## Vitamin Therapy

Check out the ingredients in Chapter 15 of the Daily Advantage Vitamin Package from Dr. David Williams. These are the highest quality money can buy and for that reason they are not cheap. However they come in simple to use plastic packets and contain a multitude of ingredients that would cost you much more if you assembled them as individual products. They are in easy to swallow capsule powder form so that they can be assimilated into the system and won't rattle around undigested for hours in your stomach.

You can only order these on line and if you sign up for Dr. Williams free monthly newsletter which contains a multitude of up to the minute health facts, you will be offered discount prices that far outweigh any store bought vitamins. Start this daily regimen today and start building your vital strength. You can order them from Mountain Home Nutritionals at 800-888-1415 or on line at www.drdavidwilliams.com

Vitamin C and Vitamin K3:

There are many Alternative Health Clinics now giving this treatment. High doses of C, up to 75 or 100 grams, (that's 100,000 milligrams, when a normal daily dose would be 2 to 3,000 milligrams). It is a powerful adjunct to the immune system, a potent antioxidant and a vital booster of the body's natural ability to kill cancer cells.

This unique combination has a synergistic effect in inhibiting the growth of breast cancer cells, and when used in conjunction with chemotherapy, increases the inhibition of cancer growth by three to four times. The anti tumor action of Vitamin K has been under investigation since 1947 when it was found to increase the effectiveness of radiation treatments and extend the longevity in patients with inoperable lung cancer. Vitamin K without the use of chemotherapy or radiation has also shown anti-cancer effects in a number of cell cultures and animal studies.

Vitamin D3 :

This is an essential supplement for anybody dealing with cancers but especially breast cancer for healing and as a preventative. Recent studies in Canada say breast cancer could be eradicated with adequate levels of this important vitamin in a woman's system; (Dr Cedric Garland at the 2010 Toronto School of Medicine Conference on Vitamin D deficiency) . 5/6000 IU a day

## Co-Q 10:

Top anti oxidant and immune/energy booster. 100 to 200 mg a day

## Iodine.

Check your levels of Iodine. You will need 12.5 mg a day. If you have cancer you will need all three of these powerful anti-oxidants and cancer fighters.

*See the list of additional nutritional supplements in Chapter 16

## Green Barley Powder

Organic Barley seed is planted and the young green shoots are harvested and freeze-dried to preserve the nutrients. The resulting powder or pill form contains all 3000 enzymes that exist in your body. Yes all 3000! And they're chockfull of chlorophyll, too, which helps your body alkalinize. The importance of keeping your body in an alkaline state cannot be over emphasized and the best way to do this is to eat greens. Green barley powder has contributed to many accounts of cancer recovery just by itself.

For more information go to www.AimInternatinal.com, where you can buy the powder or.www.GreenSupreme.net, another source for the pills. Be sure to take enough of it. They recommend up to 6 tablespoons a day or up to 20 of the pills. You can add the powder to your smoothie or dilute it in water or juice as it is quite bitter to the taste.

# Padma Basic

The Tibetan herbal formula manufactured in this country by www.econeu-genics.com is an essential part of the cancer patients recovery kit. By sealing off healthy cells this natural medicine will help prevent metastasis of cancer cells to other parts of the body while you are getting the body healthy again. Make this a daily regimine. Take up to 6 tablets per day.

# Turmeric

This miracle herb with the magical ingredient of Curcumin should be used in cooking everyday. Then also take 2 teaspoons two times a day in 1 cup of water and add a few shakes of black pepper for better assimilation. You can add it to the Green Barley Powder and take them together. If this is distasteful to your palate, use the capsules and take three in the morning and three in the afternoon with water.

# Laetrile

Apricot kernels are the cheapest form of this remedy. They come in 1lb bags for as little as $14. Grind them up and sprinkle on food. Start with two a day and work up to 10. If you become nauseous back off the dose until you build a tolerance. Amygdalin/B17 is another form of laetrile in a tablet. Both are available on line at www.apricotpower.com 1-866-468-7487. Read the book World without Cancer : The Story of B17 by G. Edward Griffin and Apricot Power : How Laetrile Cured My Cancer by Helen M. Curran.

# Hydrate

In his book Your Body's Many Cries for Water, F. Batmanghelidj M.D, finds that dehydration leads to stress and most of the chronic, degenerative diseases prevalent in our country. The simple act of consuming 8 to 10 glasses of water per day will keep you healthy better than any medications.

The cancer patient particularly needs to drink at least two glasses of room temperature water on awaking to help flush the detritus accumulated from the body's nightly cleansing. Then drink two glasses between meals but none within 2 hrs of bedtime. If you wake in the night feeling dehydrated drink another glass. Make sure the kidneys are working properly and eliminating the water you consume. Use the Sole salt water solution and add a tablespoon to your quart container every day. This helps alkalinize the body and increases the cells' ability to absorb the water. Alternatively, for a refreshing taste and healthy herbal infusion, you can add fresh lemon balm, mint and yarrow from the garden.

# Juice For Life

Get a juicer! What kind? It doesn't matter! Get a juicer! Start juicing every day. I used an old Champion for years but it is slow. Then I got the Jack Lelane centrifugal juicer which was fast and easy to clean. My recommendation for up to the minute state of the art is the Hurom Slow Juicer available through www.naturalnews.com.

Juicing fresh fruits and vegetables daily is a must to build healthy cells and blood. Choose what is in season. Green drinks which include leafy greens such as kale, collards, chard and cilantro are potent anti-oxidants. Use a carrot, apple, lemon, ginger combination for beta carotene. I do not recommend too many fruits as they are loaded with sugars and the body needs to alkalinize. Stick with fresh veggies.

# Exercise

To Get Inside-Get Outside! Every day get outside in nature if possible. Walk ten minutes from your home and walk back. Get a dog and take it for walks! They are wonderful companions when you are feeling sick and they will love you unconditionally and support your healing.

Work Out: If you are strong enough, start going to the gym regularly. Get a trainer to show you the best exercises for your condition and build up slowly. You will be amazed at how good you can feel when you tone the muscles and work the cardiovascular system. The inexpensive way to build muscle is to buy a couple of 5, 10 or 15 lb dumbbells . Do multiple repetitions using arm curls and overhead presses every morning for ten minutes. You will see your physique develop and build stamina.

Move The Lymph : The Rebounder trampoline is the single most helpful piece of exercise equipment you can own. Creating a healthy lymphatic system is essential to cleansing and rejuvenating the body. The bouncing action makes thousands of tiny valves in the lymph channels open and close rapidly. This helps to flush out toxins and deliver vital plasma where it is needed. Learn the exercises and do at least ten minutes a day. If you are too weak just do the 'Health Bounce' and bounce gently without lifting your feet off the surface of the mat.

Don't stint on this equipment. There are many brands on the market and the cheap ones do not hold up. For a lifetime warranty on parts and a piece of equipment that will accommodate years of extra duty go to www.reboundair. com. They cost around $200 plus shipping.

Join a gym, walk, jog, run, hike, do whatever it takes to get your cardiovascular system moving regularly and you will promote healing and vitality.

Yoga and Breath : This traditional Eastern discipline is so main stream, you can find classes in every town in America. Sign up for a course and go once or twice a week. Learn to do these strengthening and rejuvenating exercises at home every morning to rebuild muscle and tone. Always remember to breathe deeply to help build lung capacity, oxygenate the cardio-vascular system and bring clarity of mind. See the instructions for alternate nostril breathing under the heading Meditation, Yoga and Pranayama in the Ayurveda section of this book

# Cleanse

The importance of cleansing the body for the cancer patient cannot be overstated. There are many ways to do this and it will vary in each individual case based upon their unique situation.

I highly recommend the Ayurvedic system of *Pancha Karma* discussed in Part IV of this book. Check out travel to India or find an Ayurvedic Center near you for a consultation.

The Gerson Therapy in Tijuana, Mexico, focusing on raw food and juices, may be appropriate in your case or you may choose to do your own home based version including fasting, juicing, enemas, liver and kidney flushes. What you do and how you do it is up to you but I also highly recommend consulting an Alternative Healthcare Professional to guide you through the many stages based on your state of health. They can be there for you to answer questions and monitor your progress if you are unfamiliar with this process.

The number one thing you can do to start your program is the liver and gall-bladder flush. You can do it at home and the cost is minimal but the pay off is enormous in restoring your health. Also do a kidney cleanse by drinking the tea as outlined in Part II.

Be sure and clean the colon with the coffee enemas and the colema colonics. This way you are not starting with a clogged system as you begin to detox and add purified food and juices to your system.

After all, you wouldn't add clean oil to your car engine without first draining off the old oil!

# Bodywork

In order to facilitate you body's journey back to health, it will need caring for by skilled bodywork practitioners. Touch is a vital part of healing and your body will respond faster when it can release physically and emotionally the toxins that are being eliminated daily through cleansing practices and eating an eliminating diet. The following is a partial list of bodywork available and I recommend getting at least one of them once a week.

Lymph Drainage: This is a specialized massage technique, using light to medium pressure strokes by the therapist. The massage strokes trace the flow of the lymph system, just under the skins surface, and help to break up toxins and move them out of the body. *This type of massage is NOT suitable for women with cancer in the lymph nodes* .

Cranial Sacral: Usually performed on a person wearing loose clothes while laying on their back on a massage table. The skilled therapist works on the occipital ridge and various points on the neck and skull, all the way down the body to the feet using a light touch. The intention is to listen to the innate rhythm of the cerebral-spinal fluid as it flows up and down the body. When blockages to this flow are removed, energy can move more freely, relieving pain and soreness in muscles and fascia.

Acupuncture and Acupressure: Accupuncture is and offshoot of Traditional Chinese Medicine (TCM). It uses very fine needles inserted lightly into the top layers of the skin. These needles trace the invisible meridian lines that represent the energy flows of the body. By connecting these points, blockages are removed and pain is relieved so that healing can take place.

Accupressure does the same thing without the use of needles. By applying finger pressure to these points muscle can relax and healing energy begin to flow again.

Reflexology: This form of massage is usually applied to the feet with finger and thumb pressure. It can be deeply relaxing. Every part of the sole of the foot corresponds to an organ, or an area of the body. By applying pressure and rubbing on the the respective area pain can be relieved and toxins are removed from the area.

Reiki: This is originally a Japanese form of energy work or palm healing. The practitioner uses their hands and intention to bring healing to any part of the body. There is also a method of distance healing using special symbols.

Reichian Breathwork: This was developed in the early 1900's by scientist and psychologist, Willhelm Reich. It involves the mind and body through specific breathing techniques to release repressed emotion held in the body's muscular system. You can read more in the section on 'The Cancer Cure Pioneers.'

Osteopathy: This is a hands-on healing technique developed and first practiced by A.T.Still in 1874. It emphasizes the inter-relationship between structure and function and recognizes the body's innate ability to heal itself. The practitioner works in micro movements to help the body re-align itself. It is one of the oldest healing techniques in use today.

As with any bodywork, but specifically with Lymphatic Drainage, be prepared for emotional content to arise. Give yourself the time off following massage or bodywork and allow time to process any old, stuck emotions that may arise. They need to be honored and released.

## Diet

This is the simple key to prevention and recovery and I recommend an Ayurvedic approach. Check out the charts at the end of the book to determine your *prakruti*,(constitution), or see an Ayurvedic practitioner near you for counseling. Start implementing the right diet for you and eat the fruits and vegetables that are in season at regular mealtimes during the day.

Good digestion is the fundamental principle of good health, so no matter what cancer you are dealing with you need to regulate this important biological function. From here you may add vegetable juices and food supplements and other dietary needs as they arise.

Be serious about getting large doses of dark leafy greens and cruciferous veggies daily. Steam or stir fry them with every meal. Eliminate red meat. Stick to fish and organic chicken for your protein 2 or 3 times a week. Discover the golden grains like brown or basmati rice, quinoa (pronounced *keenwah*), millet, buckwheat, oats and barley. Use turmeric, garlic and ginger liberally. Eat all organic. Don't snack on junk! And eliminate coffee and substitute green and herbal teas.

It will depend very much on your particular state of health and your cancer diagnosis just how radical your diet has to be to achieve results. With a cancer diagnosis it is best to become strictly vegetarian and increase your ratio of raw foods and juices to stop the cancerous process and reverse the situation. This has to be a decision made between you and your health practitioners based on the evidence at hand and your gut feeling about what your body needs to begin its recovery.

## Meditate

Slow down. Find time to get quite and listen for the silence that is behind the incessant thoughts and the fear that may be arising at this time. You are more than what you look like. Much more than the body you inhabit and the world of identity. This is a time for reflection and paying attention to your intuition which will tell you the next obvious thing to do. Trust it!

# ONE MORE THING

You may want to add your own food discoveries and any of the supplements and foods in the previous chapters but remember, the most important thing is your attitude. Create a positive atmosphere amongst the people around you. Move forward in your search for the right therapy for you, whether it is all alternative or an integrative approach. Be kind to yourself and others and find something to be grateful for each day. Whenever you are feeling sad (or happy), remember to take in a deep, full breath. It will always bring you back to presence.

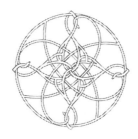

# CHAPTER 25

# YESES AND KNOWS

**H**ERE are the obvious Do's and Don'ts to promote good health but especially if you are fighting cancer. Make a copy and attach it to the refrigerator where you can see it every day. You may not be able to do all the good things every day but do as many as you can and you will see an improvement in your health. Instead of No's, which tends toward the negative, I use the word kNOw because your inner intelligence *KNOWS* that cutting out these things will move you in the right direction.

## THE YESES

- TAKE YOUR TURMERIC – 2 tsp in 1 cup water 2x a day. Add a dash of fresh ground pepper.
- BECOME ITALIAN – Eat garlic every day. Peel 'em yourself.
- SUNDRENCH WITH VITAMIN D 3– 4,000 to 5,000 mg once a day
- IODINE LOAD– Check your levels and if they are low take 50 mg per day. Test again in 3 months.
- EAT LEAFY GREENS EVERYDAY - Kale, Chard, Collards,

Mustard, Bok Choy, Cabbage, Broccoli, Dandelion, and anything with a green tint.

- SUPPLEMENT – Take your daily Vitamins especially Vitamin D 3.

- JUMP FOR JOY – Rebound on a trampoline every day for lymph health

- HYDRATE FOR HEALTH – Drink three glasses of water every morning upon arising and 6 to 8 glasses through out the day. It's Free!

- BEEKIND TO YOURSELF – Pollinate! 1 tsp of fresh bee pollen every day.

- FOCUS ON THE ROAD AHEAD – Don't look down!

- DO THE NEXT OBVIOUS THING – Get still and you will know what to do.

- ASK FOR SUPPORT – Call on your friends and family.

- BE PRO-ACTIVE – Surround yourself with POSITIVE people and ideas.

- ENTERTAIN YOURSELF – Watch funny movies, play golf, garden, read a good book. Do the things you love.

- DO THE 'SOMEDAY' THINGS – Take a trip to Hawaii!

- GET OUTSIDE! – Be in nature, see how it lives.

- BE A BEACH BUM – Go to the ocean, breathe the air, walk the shore.

- SUN GAZE – First hour of sunrise, last hour of sunset. It's Free!

- EARLY TO BED, EARLY TO RISE – 2 hours before midnight is worth 4 hours after midnight. Help the body rejuvenate.

- MEDITATE – Everyday at least 15 minutes. It will bring clarity and peace into your life.

- JUICE for life. Buy a juicer and use it every day.

- ADOPT A DOG – They are in charge of smiles. It will bring love and joy into your life.
- STICK WTH IT and you will get through this.

And finally,

- <u>CLEANSE! CLEANSE! CLEANSE!</u>

# THE KNOWS

This is what you have to eliminate if you are serious about getting well. You K(no)w this!

- ALL SUGAR – In anything, Period!
- ALCOHOL – Give it up for now. It's not for ever.
- CAFFEINE – Replace coffee and black tea with Green Tea.
- TOBACCO – Cold turkey!
- SODAS – 8 teaspoons of sugar in every can.
- DIET SODAS – Cancer causing chemicals in every can.
- JUNK FOOD – If you can't understand the ingredients on the label, you don't need them in your body.
- FAST FOOD – Eat home cooked food; SLOWLY!
- THE DAILY NEWS – TV, newspapers, magazines, internet. Face it, we are addicted to this stuff, it's mostly negative and it adds stress to our lives.
- NEGATIVE PEOPLE – Choose the opposite.
- THE TELEPHONE – Don't repeat your story over and over. Have someone else field the calls or leave a message that you are resting and tell them to send letters and cards. And get rid of your cell phone.

- BEING A VICTIM – Don't ask "Why me?" There is a lesson here. Discover the cause, remove it and get on the program!

# PART IV

# THE SOUL

*"The well is there for all. No one is forbidden to take water from it. No matter how many come, all find what they need, for the well is dependable. It has a spring and never runs dry. Therefore it is a great blessing to the whole land. The same is true of the really great man, whose inner wealth is inexhaustible; the more the people draw from him, the greater his wealth becomes."*

The I Ching or Book of Changes

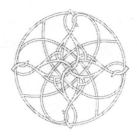

# CHAPTER 26

# THE NEW MEDICINE

*"In essence every disease should be understood as an*
*evolutionary meaningful biological program of nature.*
*In other words, every disease presents a specific program*
*that solves an exceptional, unanticipated biological conflict.*
*It is a new way of looking at disease as a significant biological*
*program of nature interpreted through the evolution of the species."*

Dr. Ryke Geerd Hamer
German New Medicine

S IMPLY put, what has come to be known as "New Medicine", is the
premise that underlying all disease is an emotional conflict, the resolution of which will result in the healing of the disease.

It is true that healing begins when diet and lifestyle are balanced and nutritional supplementation, herbal remedies and cleansing are implemented, but
we must also address the cause. In most cases this has an emotional compo-
nent-the key to which is at the core of healing.

Dr. Geert Hamer coined the term 'German New Medicine'. www.german-
newmedicine.com . In Germany, in the 1980's, he began extensive research
into his newly evolving theories. He examined thousands of his patients with
various diseases and took CT scans of their brains during the active phase

of their illness. He discovered a small growth in the cerebellum that would appear in different places but would always correspond biologically to the exact organ or limb where the disease appeared. It was as if the brain was sending a message to the body to develop a cancerous tumor that was the body's best chance of survival to relieve the unbearable stress of an emotional trauma that was influencing the patient.

Without fail, all his patients had received an emotional shock or trauma such as the death of a loved one, an accident or a severe emotional incident. Often they had been under long term psychological stress in a relationship, or life experience, that had become intolerable to them, sometimes going back years to early childhood.

Invariably, when the key to the emotional conflict was brought to light and a resolution to the trauma was found by healing the original cause, the brain acted like an electrical breaker and switched off the signal for the disease to continue. The growth in the brain would shrink and disappear and, as a result, the body would spontaneously begin the process of healing itself.

Dr Hamer's original theories have since been tested and developed in the work of Claude Sabbah in France and Gilbert Renaud in Canada through a work they call Total Biology. In "The Total Biology of the Living Creatures", Gilbert Renaud lays out the correlation between emotional trauma and the biological response of the body in any number of specific diseases including MS, osteoporosis, stroke, cancer, asthma and even the common flu. He also developed a process called Biological deprogramming to help uncover the emotional conflict. He gives workshops in the US several times a year. Find out more at www.totalbiology.com.

When the emotional body, i.e the entire collection of your thoughts, feelings, memories and reactions to stress and conflict is disturbed, out of balance and in pain, it will often crystallize as a physical symptom in the body.

To heal cancer much work must be done to uncover this emotional wounding. Anger, resentment, hate, jealousy, greed, fear, doubt, overwhelming anxiety are all expressions of a disconnection from soul or the true authentic self. Unworthiness and the basic inability to love oneself is always at the core of these feelings. The first essential aspect of healing physical disease is to have compassion for oneself and to look deeply into the cause of any emotional pain and learn to release it. Forgive yourself and forgive others for any mistakes or abuses that may have happened.

Studies have shown that when people have genuine self esteem, their ability to love others and experience joy in life increases. Spontaneous healing can and does occur when we say yes to life and endeavor to live positively with love in our hearts, fulfilling our desires and being grateful for every blessed day we are given. I believe this is why we have been born on this earth at this time .This "New Medicine" is actually as ancient as human life on earth; only we have forgotten how to incorporate it into our daily lives. It determines our every choice in how we live, what we eat to sustain optimal health, and how we treat others and ourselves. Making these intelligent choices is up to us, the rest is Grace.

When we give up the need to defend our positions and be right all the time, we surrender to what is. This doesn't mean being abused or accepting intolerable situations. It means moving in the direction of right action and least resistance, taking care of ourselves and our environment. The power to heal always comes from within by listening to our body's needs. By tapping into this *source* we can find the key element of the New Medicine and live with optimal health, vitality and love.

Permit me to ask you a question. What is the meaning of *your* life? What are you doing that makes your life worth living? If you have cancer, how has it changed your perspective on life? To recover from illness we must ask these questions in order to address our underlying discomfort. You see, in my 40 yrs of studying the deeper meanings of human existence, I believe that we are not separate from all other sentient beings. We all have that innate inner divinity that makes us all one consciousness.

We do not generally experience this in our day to day lives because we have fallen under the spell of the separate ego, which was conditioned into us by the culture and circumstances that shaped our early childhood. We struggle to survive and protect ourselves from hurt and pain believing that bad things could happen to us which, in turn, creates fear, doubt, and mistrust in everything, and towards everyone around us.

Now consider this idea, which lies at the heart of one of the world's major religions. In the period between death and re-birth the soul or the very spirit consciousness of your Being may be given the opportunity to review the lessons of the previous life in a body. It will choose what probable events will occur (karma) in the next incarnation. This includes choosing two incarnate souls to be our parents in our new human birth. In this new life we begin again to evolve as souls inhabiting a physical body without conscious remembrance of previous lifetimes. All the karma (past actions), lessons and behaviors of the previous incarnation, are carried over to work through again. This is called 'burning off' karma.

All manifestation of life on earth is an expression of the Divine Consciousness evolving moment to moment and arising spontaneously. It is unfolding effortlessly and coordinating synchronistically with everything in existence. We are at once subject to destiny *and* free will, meaning, we create our own reality and, with awareness of this knowledge, have the ability to shape our lives to varying degrees.

If you are experiencing any disease, it is a physical symptom of a much deeper emotional and spiritual imbalance. It is a tenet of every ancient spiritual teaching that the physical body has several invisible energy bodies or ***sheaths*** that emanate out from the physical body in 'layers'. When disease manifests in the physical plane it is primarily because of an imbalance in these layers caused by present lifetime emotional and psychological stress and sometimes past life karma. Understanding and accepting this, one can then make healing the core emotional issues of one's life the first priority, addressing the cause in the physical cry for help that is cancer. Without this essential work, long term healing will always be ineffective.

The world is a chaotic play of consciousness with billions of egos playing out their roles in the evolution of the earth. Wars, famine, genocide, earthquakes and natural disasters, unjust heinous crimes, are all tragedies only if they are viewed as 'bad'. In the light of non-dual consciousness and the play of opposites there is no good or bad, only what is. Every moment and every event is seen as the perfect unfolding of the Universal Divine Consciousness.

If you could look back on many of the events in your life, or the world in general, from the conscious perspective of non-egoic acceptance, you would see the dynamic unfolding of life in all its perfect brilliance. This includes everything, from the daily birth and death of humanity on the planet, to the serene and natural appearance, and disappearance, of a flower in your garden. No right, no wrong, no black, no white, no good, no bad, only now, *only this!*

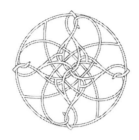

# CHAPTER 27

# WE ARE SPIRIT
## The Story of Bobsy's Return

THE music had suddenly changed. It was a cassette tape of operatic arias set to a modern beat. My son Gabriel had made it for my beloved wife Bobsy to listen to in the last days of her life. She had passed away in the next room, only 36 hours before, after less than a years struggle with cancer. It was playing now as I walked into the living room to find out who had put it on.

Willow and Bhavananda, Bobsy's two women friends who had been there at the end, were in the kitchen and bathroom helping me clean the house after all the family had left the day before. I had put on some quiet CD's to play while we cleaned up, and I was throwing out dozens of medicines from the refrigerator, when I noticed the stereo system changed to the cassette tape of operatic arias. Memories of Bobsy came flooding back to me.

I called to the two friends to join me standing in front of the music system and asked if either of them had changed the CD player to the tape player. They had both been pre-occupied with their work and hadn't noticed the change. "This was her favorite music," I said, " and I didn't put it on!" At that moment we all got a strong feeling that someone else was present in the room and we looked at each other with wide eyes. The aria seemed to increase in volume and intensity and I became chilled with goose bumps and began to feel unsteady on my legs. We all looked around the room and Bhavananda said what we were all feeling, "She's here now! Bobsy's Spirit has come back. Can you feel her in the room with us?"

To this day almost ten years later, I can still remember vividly what happened next. A feeling of absolute peace and love descended on us and pervaded the whole room. The three of us moved to the couch and chairs and were immediately overwhelmed with a palpable, blissful energy that flooded all our bodies simultaneously. My heart felt so full of joy that I began to weep uncontrollably. It was then that Bobsy began to speak telepathically to us.

"I'm alright now," she said. Her words came spontaneously into our minds as though by thought transference, but as clear as day. "I am on the other side," she went on, "and I want to tell you not be afraid, because death is just the beginning of life."

The music continued to soar and although my eyes were closed it was as though she was dancing around the room. I sensed her Spirit move close and I literally felt her embrace me as she told me she would always love me and I wept freely the tears that I had kept bottled up for the long months of her illness.

The three of us sat together in this blissful state for 45 minutes as the tape played to the end and began again. Eventually the intense feeling of blissful presence lifted and we opened our eyes and gazed incredulously at each other. We stopped the tape and made a pot of tea and sat together relating how we each had experienced the same sensations and even the things she had said to each of us was similar. For a long time we smiled and talked and it felt like a great weight had been lifted from us and we had been shown unequivocally the immortality of the human spirit.

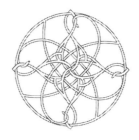

# CHAPTER 28

# EMOTIONAL HEALING

*"The journey of the Soul is to become
the purest vessel of light possible,
fully revealing that this is our true nature."*

From the book 'Luminous' by Aubrey Degnan

IN my experience there is almost always an emotional component to the cancer diagnosis, or any illness or disease in the body for that matter-because, amongst other things, the immune system is always compromised by the stresses of the mind. Call it a Spiritual crisis if you will but there can be no true healing until this emotional connection to the *dis-ease* has been thoroughly explored, understood and released. This is the premise of 'The New Medicine'.

In my own case it was connected to the grief that I was unable to hold and integrate after the loss of my dear wife to cancer. When she passed away after a year of failing slowly, I was an exhausted, inconsolable wreck. My whole world had been destroyed and I felt devastated and angry. Although I didn't know it at the time, I went into what I now see was a kind of painful emotional limbo, unable to feel the deep hurt I was experiencing with the loss of everything in the world that felt dear to me.

Years later, on a mystical, dreamlike level, I came to see it as though I had entered a dark forest, carrying my grief wrapped up tightly in a bundle close to my chest. I found a quiet glade where I dug a hole and buried the bundle of grief and covered it over with the earth. Then I walked back out of the forest to face the world again.

There were times when I would return to the forest, dig up my grief and spend some time with it. But it was so painful I would always put it back in the ground and cover it over until the next time, until eventually I rolled a large boulder on top of the hole and decided never to go back there again.

Finally, after several years of my own bout with cancer, I realized the need for the release of the anger and grief that I had buried inside myself which had probably contributed to my own illness. At some point in that discovery-and it always comes at the perfect moment for each person's unfolding on their path of life learning-I made the metaphoric journey back to the forest and was able to roll back the boulder from the hole and retrieve the grief again.

Then there was a process of un-wrapping the grief, feeling the pain of it and sitting with it until I was finally able to allow the hurt feelings into my heart to be healed. Then something wonderful happened. By welcoming the grief and allowing myself to be broken hearted, I began to accept the lessons that had been given to me in order to grow spiritually. From that acceptance came a gratitude for what I did have in life and the recognition of my connection to everything, particularly the people who had loved and cared for me through the darkest times of my illness.

This led to finding the will to live fully again, and by integrating the heart break into my soul, I was able to heal on both an emotional and physical level. I left the dark forest to return to the world feeling healed and with the desire to live and love again, and with a new awareness of people and events imbued with meaning and presence.

A diagnosis of cancer, an accident, the loss of a loved one, the end of a career or a divorce; all can seem like a death sentence from which there is no escape. Yet miraculously these apparent tragedies represent a chance for learning, for we have a chance to experience wisdom, and a depth of love, that we were not open to before the event. The remorseless journey of human activity on this planet, although sometimes appearing chaotic, unjust and unreasonable, is the incessant 'Flow of the Universe', unfolding with perfect timing in every moment. Knowing this wisdom, is the beginning of a healthy, balanced life full of joy and compassion for oneself and others.

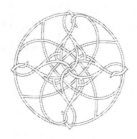

# CHAPTER 29

# THE WELCOMING PROCESS

*"Saying 'No' from the bottom of your heart, is truly saying 'Yes' to yourself"*
From the book 'The Art of Selflove'
by Frank M. Lobsiger.

THERE was a period in my recovery when I was going through a very difficult time and I was filled with anxiety and the fear of death. I was at a healing crossroads and didn't know where to turn for a way out of the symptoms I was experiencing. Every night I was unable to sleep and I would wake bathed in sweat with the sheets soaked through. Although I was unaware of it at the time, this was a healing crisis as my body worked diligently to rid itself of the foreign invaders and eliminate the toxins through my sweat glands. I had horrendous nightmares and at times I felt like I was possessed. I was truly despairing of my recovery from cancer.

When I woke up in the dark alone and afraid I didn't know what to do, so one night I decided to call my good friend Frank to talk to him about my fears. Frank is a Somatic Therapist who lives in Switzerland, so at 3 am my time he would be awake and going about his day. The first time I called he answered the phone and suggested he try a process with me which he was developing for a book he was writing on self-love.

This simple exercise is called 'The Welcoming Process '[TM] and is in three parts. The first step is called "Welcoming" and he asked me

*"What is the content of your experience right now?"*

I described to him that I was overwhelmed with the fear of my impending death and it hung on me like a wet blanket that I couldn't shake off. Then he asked me the second step;

*"Can you allow this experience?"*

In my case he asked very specifically if I could allow the fear and the experience of dying. Having had some exposure to *allowing* deep feeling in my body, I was able to say "Yes" and I began to stop resisting the intensity of the fear and its hold on my body. If I had said "No" to the feeling, this was okay too, and Frank would have asked me if I could allow the "no" or the "resistance", so that there was never a moment of impasse. This enabled the process to flow smoothly to the next step, which was;

*"Noticing the Body Shift"*

This is when the body reacts somatically to the *actual allowing* of one's here and now experience, A physical body movement of release happens automatically. It can be very obvious, like a deep breath or yawning, or it can be more subtle with slight movements or changes in body tension. Once this is noticed and acknowledged, one returns to the 'Welcoming' step, exploring the content of one's experience in the *next* moment, and if one can allow these new feeling sensations.

As Frank worked with me that night I went through rapid changes in my feelings as he repeated the steps and I allowed, or didn't allow, the experiences. I noticed profound changes happening rapidly in my body/mind as my breathing deepened and my body jerked and trembled and the deep fears melted away. This is a simplified description of the process of course, but it was powerfully transforming for me and in less then half and hour I was completely healed of the dark negative influences that had been disturbing my sleep. My optimism and love of life returned. I felt deeply relaxed and free of fear and I actually felt hungry and wanted to get up and eat a hearty breakfast, something I hadn't done in days.

Frank was developing 'The Welcoming Process' at the time and he has since created it into a self-healing practice and incorporated this amazing technique in a book called "The Art of Selflove – Loving Yourself is the Key to Happiness". You can find this wonderful book on his website at www. theartofselflove.com

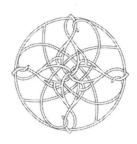

# CHAPTER 30

# THE HEALING POWER OF DREAMS, VISIONS AND SOUNDS

*"There is only one thing that we can control in the human life,*
*and that one thing is not our mind.*
*It's not a thought, it's not our breath,*
*it's not our responses, it's not our actions.*
*It is the cultivation of personal awareness,*
*the moment-to-moment awareness of*
*who we are – in charge of our life,*
*in charge of our purpose, in charge of our path."*

Mother Maya

## Dreams

EARLY in the process of my recovery from cancer, I had a dream that revealed to me a path of emotional release and also a vision of the very woman, who I would eventually find in real life, to help guide me in how to do it.

In the dream I was in a large dance studio with a wooden floor. There were various men and women dancing together practicing a form of "contact improvisation" whereby each partner learns to lift and roll with each other in a fluid dance like motion to the rhythm of the music.

There was a woman instructor in dance attire moving around the studio giving instruction. I was turned on by the dance groups and sat down on the side to watch her instruct a powerfully built , muscular man dancing with two women. As the man lay on his back and lifted the two women, one on each arm like pushing up weights, the woman instructor leaned over on her hands and knees and gently blew on his face. Immediately the man lost his power and the two women fell to the floor. The man began to shrink and shrivel up until in no time at all he became a tiny baby wriggling happily on its back on the dance floor.

I was amazed by this sudden transformation and leaned over to the woman and inquired what this process was called. She turned her head to look at me and replied that it was called 'Reichian Breathwork'. As soon as she spoke these words my body was transfused with an electric energy that began to shake me from head to toe with glorious waves of sexual ecstasy. At that moment I woke up in bed in the middle of a deep, inner orgasm and my pelvis was jerking uncontrollably with pleasurable sexual energy.

The dream was so powerful that I wrote it down right then and there, and resolved to find out what Reichian Breathwork was all about. Over the next few days I researched on the internet and began to read about Wilhelm Reich, an Austrian Psychologist and Scientist and one time student of Sigmund Freud, who had developed theories about healing the human psyche using breathing techniques to release buried emotions held in the musculature armor of the body.

I asked friends if they knew of anybody who did this work in the Santa Cruz area but none came to light. A few weeks later I was visiting a doctor in Western Sonoma near Santa Rosa a few hours north of where I lived. I was flip-ping through the local free weekly, newspaper in his reception area and there, on the inside back page, was a large advertisement that said 'REICHIAN BREATHWORK' accompanied by a picture of the woman instructor I had seen in my dream. With my heart racing, I whipped out my cell phone and called the phone number in the advertisement. The woman answered and I told her she had appeared in a dream I had had about Reichian Breathwork and that I wanted to learn more about her work. There was an opening available in a few days.

What followed was an extraordinary journey of emotionally freeing breathing sessions over a period of 2 years that profoundly affected my recovery from cancer and began to reveal to me the mind/body, emotional/spiritual component of illness, and the importance of revealing its hidden meaning, which is at *the heart of all true healing.*

Dreams can provide information from the deep sub-conscious mind. Whatever is not acknowledged in the waking state, and especially if it is an emotional issue, it may be turned into a dream with symbolic characters and objects that can reveal some information for you to process and understand.

Keep a journal by your bed and if you wake in the night with the memory of a dream that seems important, write it down, or at the very least jot down a key phrase that will jog your memory in the morning. Here is an example of a dream that told me very specifically what I had been doing in my own life up until the cancer struck.

In the dream I appeared as a young boy with a pet bird in a small cage. I knew I loved the bird dearly and yet when I took a close look at it I noticed that it was lying on the bottom of the cage with its beak crushed and it's feathers molting and in disarray. I was mortified to see my pet in this state and began to weep uncontrollably. I opened the cage door and held the bird in the palm of my hand where upon it magically changed and looked perfectly healthy and normal. Then it flew off into the sky and I felt a profound sense of relief.

I interpreted the dream to mean that as a child I had closed down my heart and I had been ignoring my Soul's desires for most of my life. The bird represented my Spirit trapped inside my body, dying from lack of attention and love. I will never forget the feeling of sorrow and regret I felt upon awaking from that dream and I resolved from that day forth to begin to open my heart and set my Spirit free.

## Asking For A Dream

Here is a way to stimulate your ability to have dreams that will guide you in your healing. Just before going to sleep say the following phrase to yourself quietly, "Please give me a dream I can ___remember and understand___." Focus on a question or subject where you want more clarity. Imagine a blue light in the area of your throat as you fall asleep. This is the 5th chakra and gives voice to creative expression. When recovering from cancer, dreams can be powerful healing tools that speak to your heart and even provide you with solutions and answers to situations that have been hidden from your conscious thought.

## Visions

Similar to dreams, visions have the ability to guide you on your path to wellness and can provide you with insight and direction. You can initiate a vision by doing a guided Shamanic "journey." This journey may be facilitated by a guide who will talk you through it, often with the accompaniment of a drum or rattle to help you drop into a trance state. Or you may simply lay on the floor or the bed and with the help of some trance like music you can take yourself on a vision quest to find answers to your life situation or healing path.

The journey always starts with you mentally going to a place in nature in your imagination. From there you will look for a hole or fissure in the earth which might be a cave or tunnel often with steps leading down. Once you enter this hole and begin the descent anything can happen, and you may meet a guide in the form of a person or more often than not an animal. After your adventure in the dream world, when certain things may have been shown or told to you, you will return via the same entrance in the earth and come out of your trance or dreaming state.

One night, when I was at the very depths of hopelessness and at a stage in my illness when I didn't know if I would live or die, I decided to take a salt and soda bath. Laying there in a state of half conscious, dream-like surrender, I had the vision of the Native American Indian coming to me and telling me I was going to live, (See Chapter 10). This vision led to my determination to come out of the despair I had sunk into following the failed cancer salve experiment on my tumor.

From that day on things turned around for me. I was guided to make some phone calls which led directly to me finding a healer who would bring me from the edge of despair and infuse me with new hope. Making the choice to live is no guarantee, only a chance to go forward in a new direction.

Facing serious, life threatening illness we may all come to a place like this sooner or later and we must ask ourselves this question; do I want to live or move on at this time? Some of us will choose the former and some the latter and each choice is equally valid and each is an attempt to shift the status quo from where we are at. Only one thing is guaranteed and that is our freedom of choice. From there on, once the choice is made, we are in the hands of Grace.

## Sounds

There are many esoteric chants or mantras that are useful in creating and benefiting health and healing. I am going to give you three that are some of the most simple and powerful sounds that you can create to bring positive and effective change in your life.

1. The sound _Aaahh_ is one of the most basic and primordial sounds that humans have made for eons. To use this simple chant, find a time and place when no one will be disturbed by your sounding. Sit comfortably and begin by taking a deep breath in through the nose, and open the mouth wide to form the Aaahh shape. Let the sound come on the out breath at whatever tone, high or low, that feels comfortable to you. Extend the sound with the full exhale until you feel ready to take another breath. Don't force it, let it come naturally at its own pace..

   Breathe in again slowly and fully and release the breath again with the sound _Aaaaahhhh_ drawn out as long as is comfortable. You may vary the tone and intensity of the sound as you feel appropriate. Continue for 5 or 10 minutes and visualize a completely healthy body. This will work for anything you want to manifest in your life. If you cough or are interrupted by yawning or breathing difficulties, simply relax and begin the chant again on the next exhale. Once you practice this sound and become comfortable with it, it will take on a life or sound of its own and fill your mind and body with its energy and powerful vibration.

2. The sound _Om_ or _Aum_ is probably the most commonly used ancient chant first brought to the West by the Buddhists in the last hundred years. It is used universally to instill peace and tranquility in a gathering or personal meditation and it is extremely potent in healing and balancing energy in the body. Don't underestimate this well known chant. It really has the ability to heal and transform the very cells of the body with its vibrational power.

   When sitting comfortably one can begin with the chin slightly tucked and then take a deep belly/chest breath and exhale with the mouth shaped to make an _aahhooo_ sound. Slowly lift the head and look up as you continue sounding the _ooooohhhh_ finally bringing the chin down again so it is slightly tucked. Maintain the _mmmmm_ vibration for as long as possible before taking another deep breath and starting again.

3. The third sound has a story attached to it. It was told to me by one of my teachers, Dr. Vasant Lad, one of the foremost Ayurvedic Physicians in the world who founded The Ayurvedic Institute in New Mexico. He told me that many years ago when he was a visiting physician at a hospital in India he was introduced to one of the patients who had an incurable disease and was only given a month to live. The man was nearly blind and could hardly swallow food or water but he asked if there was anything that Dr Lad could do for him. Dr Lad thought carefully and then suggested that during the last stages of his life at least the man could be conscious of his breath by chanting the holy phrase *So Hum,* which means *"I am That"*.

When Dr Lad revisited the hospital a month later the man was still alive and was practicing the chant continuously every day. A month after that he was still alive and repeating the So Hum chant with every breath. Six months later he was still alive. A year later he was still alive and is alive and healthy to this day.

*So Hum* is a Sanskrit word and the Sanskrit language is one of the oldest known to man, having a special healing vibration in its phonetic sounding. Many of the prayer mantras are specific ritual prayers to invoke a Spiritual Presence in the speaker and the listener. Whenever you can, sit still and say the word *So* on the in-breath and *Hum* on the out-breath. This one may be done silently in the mind and is just as powerful.

These are all easy sounds to learn and use to heal illness in the body. Take the time first thing in the morning before or after meditation or throughout the day to ground yourself with these sounds. When fear arises about your diagnosis and you feel overwhelmed, remember Dr Lads' story. Repeat *So Hum* with your next breath, and your next breath.

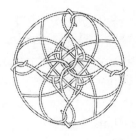

CHAPTER 31

# ALL THAT EXISTS

*"This moment..., wonderful moment!"*
Thich Nhat Hanh

ONCE upon a time, long ago, in a far away kingdom, there lived a king who was fabulously wealthy. He had everything he could wish for but he often became morose and fell into deep states of depression. He decided one day to call upon the wise men of his country to find an answer to his sadness.

Eventually one wise old monk showed up at the palace and asked for an audience with the king. The king asked him why it was that with all his wealth and possessions that he was often unhappy. The monk told him that to find the answer to this question would cost a great deal. The king assured him he would spare no cost to find the answer to his problem. The wise monk replied that it would take more than all the wealth the king possessed but that he would go away and return with an answer in three weeks.

The monk returned on the appointed day and brought with him an exquisitely carved box made of precious jade. He gave it to the king and told him the answer to his question lay within. Opening the box carefully the king saw that it contained a golden ring. On the circle of the ring inscribed in silver was an inscription. It said *"All That Exists Passes Away...This I Know."*

The monk then told the king to wear the ring always and the next time he was feeling depressed about something, or feeling sorry for himself, he should look at the ring and read the inscription knowing that his state of unhappiness was only temporary. Further more, whenever he was feeling happy, he should remember to look at the ring and read the inscription and know that this mood too would pass. This would help him remember the transitory nature of things and he would not get stuck in any mood for long ever again.

When we are sick, symptoms can arise out of nowhere accompanied by many moods of fear and doubt and the eventuality of death. As in the story above, know that these symptoms and fears will eventually change and pass and new feelings will replace them. Even when we wake up free of pain and sickness and feel optimistic about our health, be grateful for that day, that moment. Enjoy it and know that it is also temporary and ephemeral. We are mortal and our time here is fleeting when viewed in the great scheme of things. When we are taking our last breath, all the riches in the world will mean nothing to us.

Remember that the body is a barometer of the minds' thoughts. Try and keep your thoughts as positive as possible knowing that moods change with every passing hour. If you find it difficult to break out of a depression, feel into it deeply and try to allow the emotions to come to the surface without judging them. Take deep, slow breaths and practice the 'Welcoming Process' described in chapter 29 of this book.

Many people have been profoundly changed by a diagnosis of cancer. Some even say that it was a blessing in disguise because it showed them the fragility of life and made them grateful to be alive and appreciate health again. Remember the *"attitude of gratitude"* and use the affirmation, *"Everyday in everyway I am grateful for my healing."* Ask yourself what other things you are grateful for in your life. And remember to take life one day at a time.

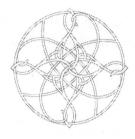

CHAPTER 32

# WE DON'T KNOW

*".....relax into the moment and let the universe do the driving.*
*If there were a secret to happiness in life,*
*I'd say this was it."*

Jed McKenna
From the book, 'Spiritual Enlightenment: The Damnest Thing'

**Y**EARS ago, when the retreat center Tassajara was being built in the California coastal mountains, the founder and teacher Suzuki Roshi had set a task for some of the monks on retreat there. He was an inveterate collector of rocks, which he liked to arrange in an aesthetic and beautiful way so that they blended in perfectly with the surrounding landscape. He had noticed a particularly large round boulder in the middle of the small creek which ran through the property. During the retreat there was a work period when the monks would be assigned a task to perform silently and consciously, such as cleaning, cooking, or working on the grounds to help their practice and also support the general functioning of the community. Early in the retreat he asked for six volunteers to go to the creek, dig out this big rock and bring it back up to the main garden.

On the first day the group assigned the task studied the rock and began to remove smaller stones around it. As they exposed more of the rock, it appeared that a large part of it was buried in the creek bed, and it was much bigger than they had first realized. Several days passed and Suzuki asked how they were

209

progressing. Not wanting to disappoint their teacher, they informed him they would soon have the rock available for him. However, with each work period, as they exposed more of the rock, it became clear that the task was proving more difficult than it had first appeared.

Finally, on about the 6th day, Suzuki said that he would come to the creek to help them. On this day, like the previous ones, they all hiked up their monk's robes and waded into the creek armed with shovels and pry bars and began to try to move the rock. Now this was a silent retreat, so all the work progressed in silence as each monk worked diligently in the water encircling the rock and all that could be heard was the clinking of shovels and the occasional effortful grunting.

While all this was happening, a member of the public, out on a hike, was crossing the wooden bridge over the creek just above where Suzuki and the monks were working. The hiker stopped in the middle of the bridge to watch the monks splashing about in the creek. After some time curiosity got the better of him and he called down to them, "What are you doing?" he asked..

Without a moments hesitation Suzuki Roshi looked up and shouted back "We don't know!" This was a moment of revelation for the student monks who all broke out laughing at the apparent wisdom of the remark and their own frustrations over the previous days in trying to complete a seemingly impossible task.

There is a lesson for all of us in this story. Ultimately, we don't know what will happen to us, even in the next minute, or the next hour, or day, or next month. We can make plans, but the future is a mystery, the past is a memory and all we really have is this moment. Yes! *right here, right now,* as you read these words. Just stop reading for a moment............. Take a deep breath and feel the life energy that is beating your heart.................Nowhere to go, nothing to do, and everything happens by itself.

If we are ill with a serious illness such as cancer, it has a tendency to focus the mind like nothing else. All those little tasks and everyday troubles, like bills and work, seem insignificant when facing a life threatening illness that we sometimes feel powerless over. But the phrase "We don't know" can bring us some peace here, if we allow it to sink in. We <u>don't</u> know what's going to happen to us. Yes, we are going to die some day, but we'd all like it to be later rather than sooner. It is at this crucial point, however, that we are faced with an important choice.

We can decide to work on moving the rock! Even if we are not sure that what we're doing is working. Even if we feel worse than yesterday. Even if all hope appears to be gone, we can keep diligently trying to move the immovable object. If we keep our eyes on the road ahead and our mind in the present, sometimes, "providence moves too," and small gains are made. Our attitude and our determination empower us to take the next step.

So take each day as it comes. There are no guarantees, and some of us will inevitably decide that it is time to move on. The Spirit that inhabits all of these miraculous bodies will eventually leave for the next adventure, just like thousands of us do every day.

We don't know.

# PART V

## THE SENSES

# THE AYURVEDIC LIFESTYLE

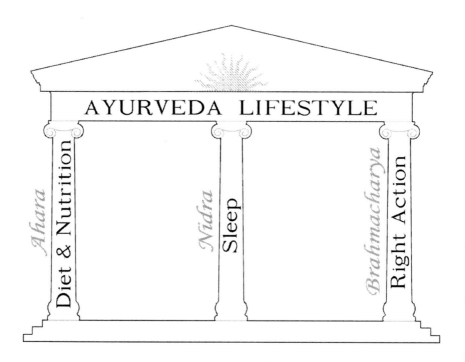

Figure 4: The Three Pillars of Ayurvedic Health

# AYURVEDA

## 'The Art of Being'

### A SHORT EXPLANATION OF A
### 5,000 YEAR OLD HEALING TRADITION

It is not my intention here to present a detailed explanation of Ayurveda. That would take a whole book in itself and there are plenty of them out there if you wish to know more. Here I want to explain a few main principles so you will understand the basic ideas behind the Ayurvedic healing methods related to any disease, including cancer.

I am not advocating Ayurveda as a complete, infallible healing system for the many types of cancer. I do, however, recommend it as the <u>foundation</u> of any recovery and reversal process to bring the body back to health and as an insurance to prevent any disease occurring again. As such it is an integral part of The Natural Cancer Recovery Program.

The following general outline is written specifically for the layperson. I have tried to keep a deep and comprehensive healing system easy to understand so that it may be quickly adopted by anyone wishing to use the program outlined in this book to recover from cancer and consider making Ayurveda a way of life.

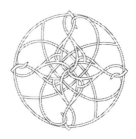

# CHAPTER 33

# THE INDIAN SYMPHONY

THE first sounds begin quietly in the morning dark, floating on the warm breeze that rustles the tall coconut palms. In the distance, amplified on the wind across the sleeping village, a soft Indian flute, rhythmic, entrancing, is followed by a woman's voice in a Sanskrit chant, high pitched and lyrical, the sweet sound of devotion. It is 5 am.

A little later the first of the morning birds, the whip-poor-will, distant and repetitive...whoopa, whoopa, whoopa, the avian alarm clock of this South Indian State. Nearby, crows join in outside my window, raucous and laughing, demanding to be heard. Next the cockerels begin their daily competition to see who is boss of the neighborhood. Soon the dogs start barking and there seems to be two or three right next door. Finally the little buses, barreling along this country lane, crammed with people hanging from the open doors. The lead footed drivers honk at any excuse with their air horns...biddly-bat! biddly-bat! biddly-bat, "get out of the way! I'm in a hurry!" It is barely 6 am and India is awake.

After my hair-raising journey from the airport by taxi, with everyone trying to overtake each other by madly honking their horns, and narrow escapes are measured in fractions of an inch, I have arrived at the SNA Ayurveda Clinic in the little village of Mannuthy in Kerala. I have come here for Pancha Karma treatment to cleanse and detox my body. This morning, as usual, breakfast arrives at 7am. Thin pancakes made from rice with a coconut milk cereal to dip them in. Delicious!

I will be here for a month and each day I have two treatments. At 10 am I am laid on a long wooden table with soft pads to support my boney body. Hot medicated oil is poured over me from little silver pots with spouts. There are four young men, two on each side and they work as one, sweeping the oil over my skin with long rhythmic strokes. I am turned on my side, then my stomach, then the other side, and then the front again until I feel like I am cooked to a turn by the warm oil.

The oil runs down the side channels of the table to a hole at the foot where it is collected in a bowl to be reheated again. There is one person to catch the oil, another to heat it and another to dab my face with a cloth if it gets splashed by the oil. There are seven people attending me and I feel like a king. Afterwards I am led to a bathroom where I pour hot water over myself from a huge basin and soap myself off. Then back to my room to rest and let the treatment 'sink in'.

It is November and the weather is a moist, tolerable 90 degrees. The tail end of the South West monsoon is just blowing through and brings with it torrential downpours. The palm trees sway and dance to the rattle of the rain on the tin roof. Suddenly the rain stops and a hot, sticky steam rises from the pavement. I walk through the small village lanes and am greeted with smiles from the families sitting outside their houses. Laughing children play in the streets unencumbered by the western addiction to an electronic screen for entertainment. Their beauty sometimes takes my breath away. I am so taken with their innocence that I find it difficult to ask them to pose for a photograph. I need not worry. Once I take my camera out, children appear from nowhere and point at themselves shouting, "Photo! photo!" They laugh and giggle when I show them the captured digital image.

In the afternoon my second treatment is called Shirodhara. It starts with me lying down on the table after an oil massage by two young men. Fresh, raw, warm milk suffused with herbs is poured slowly from a bowl suspended above my head. The milk flows evenly across my forehead and is gently massaged into my scalp. This will balance my brainwaves and calm the whole nervous system. Afterwards, a hot bath and rest before supper at seven-always fresh chapattis with spicy mung dahl. Yum!

Evening arrives and the sun settles behind the forest canopy like a smokey, orange ball. Huge hawklike bats glide through the dusk and land in the tree-tops by flipping themselves upside down to hang in the branches. The buses have returned these industrious people to their homes and all the birds are quiet, preparing to sleep. Now the crickets take the last chords of this daily symphony and some frogs join in from the lily pond in the front garden. For a few hours, India will be quiet.

After this first experience I will to return each year to India for cleansing and rejuvenation and begin to write this book. The **Pancha Karma** cleanse will become one of the most interesting and rewarding experiences of my life. This South Western part of India is alive with vibrant energy and the people are unfailingly warm and friendly. They radiate a simplicity and joy not found in the complicated lives of most Americans and this Ayurvedic experience has made me a healthier, happier and wiser human being. I am eternally grateful to India, her people and her Ayurveda.

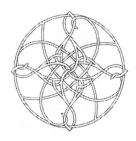

CHAPTER 34

# A QUESTION OF BALANCE

OUR world is governed by the rhythms of everyday life. The sun rises and sets, the moon waxes and wanes, the weather changes with the seasons and the ocean tides ebb and flow twice a day. All this has been happening for millions of years, day in and day out. And yet we take it for granted and often ignore the effects these natural cycles have on our lives.

Everyone's body responds to the circadian rhythms that tell us when to eat and when to sleep, when to work and when to rest. The cycles of the moon govern the weather, the growth of plants, the tidal flows and a woman's menstrual cycle. The seasons change according to the 365 revolutions of the earth around our sun each year.

We live in chaotic times, in large metropolis' powered by artificial energy and bustling with human activity. We are driven by man made schedules that push us to perform on demand to keep a shelter over our heads and food on the table. It is a far cry from our fore-fathers' times, before the discovery of fossil fuels, when humans lived in harmony with nature by gathering the fruits of the season and working the land to grow their own food.

Small wonder then that we have become alienated from these natural rhythms as we strive to keep up with the demands of a 21ˢᵗ century culture bent on an ever increasing need to accumulate and consume. We are connected to a global network of instant communication seen through computers and TV, with information overload, telling us what is happening, everywhere, all of the time. In the fast paced, fast food, instant gratification societies of the western world we have become habituated to living and eating under stress. This has led many of us away from a more balanced and relaxed way of living. We are cut off from contact with nature and unaware of the sunrise and sunset and the circling stars in the night sky. Our immune systems become weak and our bodies are vulnerable to disease and psychological trauma.

That's the bad news. The good news is that Ayurveda, the ancient, 5000 year old traditional medicine of India, has always recognized this tendency towards human imbalance and presents us with a way of bringing ourselves back into harmony with nature. *"Ayur"* means life and the word *"veda"* literally translates into knowledge or "science."

Thus an understanding of how to live a healthy life was revealed and developed by the ancient Rishis or wise men of India. Often living for many hundreds of years, these great Masters studied, refined and passed on this oral knowledge down through many generations. It was tested and adapted over thousands of years until it was written down and recorded by the first Indian physicians and surgeons in the middle ages. Its guiding principles are as true today as they were in ancient times. They now serve as a model for living that can be adopted by anyone today who wants to live a healthy, balanced life in harmony with the cycles of nature.

## CURE 'vs' HEALING

Western medicine is based on reductionism, meaning that it sees the body as a collection of parts rather than as a whole. It tries to find a cure by isolating the disease and treating the symptom as a separate problem from the person experiencing it. If the problem can be isolated and eliminated, by cutting it out (surgery), burning (radiation) or poisoning (chemotherapy), the patient should get well again. It has excellent diagnostic tools for finding the problem, but is limited in its methods of treatment, often motivated by financial gain from the large pharmaceutical and medical equipment industry. They are more interested in selling a drug or treatment to fix the problem and turn a profit, rather than providing a cure.

Ayurveda, on the other hand, is health centered. It looks first to prevent disease and sees a person experiencing a symptom as a whole person with a mind, consciousness and spirit that is temporarily out of balance. Its intent is to discover and remove the cause of the problem. It prescribes a set of diet and lifestyle changes that perhaps includes traditional herbal remedies, specifically suited to the individual, and a cleansing method called *Pancha Karma,* to detoxify the body. This not only addresses the symptoms, but begins to bring the person back into a healthy balance with nature, thereby allowing the body to heal itself.

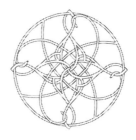

# CHAPTER 35

# THE *DOSHAS*

## (THE THREE BIOLOGICAL BODY TYPES)

AYURVEDA recognizes three different body-types, or "biological modes." Their Sanskrit names are; *Vata, Pitta* and *Kapha.* These are collectively called the *doshas.* This means that everyone has a unique set of physical needs and qualities. When a person's *dosha* is understood, it is easier to treat, feed and prescribe a lifestyle for that person, so that they can maintain optimal health through out their life.

Everyone is a combination of all three of the *doshas.* One is usually more dominant however, and sometimes two can be equally balanced, and these qualities characterize the main physical, emotional and psychological make up of that person. This constitution is set at conception by the genealogical make-up of the parents and in Sanskrit it is called the *prakruti.* This unique combination of characteristics can be discovered by reading a person's pulse and by observing their physical, emotional and psychological qualities.

In Ayurveda *everything* in the Universe is characterized by this system. Not only the body type of humans, but also for plants, animals, herbs, times of day, seasons of the year and activities performed. Furthermore, each *dosha* also contains two of the five molecular elements, i.e. Ether, Air, Fire, Water and Earth. These are the building blocks of nature, of which everything in the known Universe is comprised.

## *Vata* (Change)

Qualities : Dry, Cold, Clear, Mobile, Light, Subtle, Rough.

Elements : Ether (Space) and Air

*Vata's* are generally a thin, boney, body type with thin skin and prominent veins. The *Vata* person has the elements of air and ether (space). Talkative by nature with a nervous energy, they are hyperactive, cerebral people who have lots of ideas, but find it difficult to focus on one thing at a time. They adapt more easily than most to change. Their movements are light and quick. They are fast learners but have short memories. They dislike loud overcrowded places, often preferring the spaciousness of nature.

Being cold and dry by nature they dislike cool, damp and draughty environments preferring instead a warm, moist climate. Hawaii would be a perfect environment for them. They do best when eating a diet consisting of warm, heavy, soupy foods and casseroles that are grounding and nourishing. They occasionally need to add meat to their diet to increase their vitality and strength. They tend to skip meals and eat scantily. They really need to eat often because of a tendency toward malnourishment and low blood sugar. Their healthy tastes are sweet, sour and salty. They are poor savers and spend money quickly. Emotional by nature, they can be fearful and anxious. They do best in careers involving the creative arts, music and care giving.

They are multi-tasking, "big picture" people who have many projects happening at once and find it difficult to stick with on thing and complete it. They can have an "always on the go" nature, often over doing things and exhausting themselves physically. They would do better to rest between activities to slow themselves down.

## *Pitta* (Focus)

Qualities : Hot, Sharp, Light, Liquid, Mobile, Oily

Elements : Fire and Water

*Pitta* people are more athletic body types with a fiery, action oriented, competitive nature. Because *Pitta* is about transformation they have a strong appetite for life and can consume a lot of food at a fast pace. They have usually cleared their plates and on their way for second helpings before a *Vata* person has finished talking and taken three bites. *Pitta* people can have a sharp nature and when upset they can be cutting and critical and quick to anger. They can get irritable if they miss a meal or are overly hungry.

They are neat, focused and precise people and make good managers and entrepreneurs often preferring self-employment. Having the qualities of fire and water, they create 'steam' and generally do not like hot climates. They need to avoid hot, spicy, oily, fried foods and do best with a diet that is more focused on raw, cooling foods such as vegetables, salads and dairy and they do best with astringent, bitter and sweet tastes. Their emotional nature tends toward anger and irritability and they can be hot headed and "burn out." Their sharp, analytical nature makes them great CEO's, politicians, doctors, business owners, entrepreneurs and lawyers. They are "shoot first and ask questions later" people and tend to be the "movers and shakers" of the world.

## *Kapha* (Nourishment)

Qualities : Heavy, Slow/Dull, Cold (Damp), Oily, Slimy/Smooth, Dense, Static, Soft.

Elements : Water and Earth

*Kapha* dominant people tend to be big boned, larger in size and slower in action. Being made up of the elements of earth and water, (which creates mud) they gain weight easily and can become congested and sluggish. Their attributes are compassion, strength and stamina. They are slow to get started, but with a lot of staying power. They can over-indulge in sweet things when they feel lacking, and have an inherent dislike of exercise. They have a good memory and once a task is memorized, they have a long term ability to retain information. They are resilient and rarely get sick, but can recover quickly if they do. They are usually warm, loving, compassionate people who like to hug a lot. They may have an emotional tendency to attachment and greed. On the good side they accumulate money easily and are good savers. They prefer repetitive jobs and make good bankers, nurses, insurance agents or factory workers.

The best foods for them are warm, light and dry with astringent, bitter and sour tastes. They should avoid wheat and dairy as it can cause congestion in them. It is best for them to eat less quantity and they often like to skip breakfast and sleep in. This can cause them to feel sluggish and heavy in the morning. They need to eat their main meal at lunch and have a light evening meal three hours before going to bed – avoiding the tendency to stay up late – which will help them get up earlier in the morning. *Kapha* people tend to give selfless support and care for others and it is good for them to learn to nourish themselves.

# SUMMARY

Each *dosha* or body type has a certain diet and lifestyle that helps keep it balanced and in harmony with life. When we go against these natural principles, the quality of the *dosha,* i.e. earth, fire, water, air or ether, becomes aggravated and over stimulated. For instance *Vata* becomes spun out, overwhelmed and dried-up, as if caught in a wind storm. *Pitta* types can become angry and inflamed and burn up when their heat is increased. *Kapha* people tend to become congested with phlegm building up moisture in the lungs, causing asthma and bronchitis leading to a dull, heavy quality.

If we ignore these warning signs over time and continue living against our nature, these ailments become exacerbated. Problems deep in the tissues build up, eventually showing themselves as major diseases such as diabetes, cancer and heart attacks. Therefore it makes sense to keep optimally healthy with a diet and lifestyle that supports our particular *dosha* or biological mode, maintaining our 'balance' and living in harmony with nature.

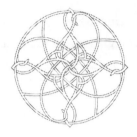

CHAPTER 36

# THE SEVEN *DHATUS*

## (THE TISSUE LAYERS OF THE BODY)

THE body is made up of skin, bone, muscles and blood, etc. These are collectively known as the "*dhatu*" tissues. In Ayurveda there are 7 tissues which support the human frame and hold everything together. They have the Sanskrit names of :

- *Rasa* ( plasma ), commonly known as the lymph; an intricate system of millions of micro channels helping to move nutrients around the body and clean up any toxic waste

- *Rakta* ( blood cells ), flowing through the arterial system from the heart and back to the lungs for re-oxygenation

- *Mamsa* ( muscle), keeping the body supple and flexible and supplying the energetic force to move the limbs

- *Meda* (adipose tissue or fat), skin absorption and elimination, insulation and support

- *Asthi* ( bone ), forming the basic skeletal structure of the body supporting the skin, muscles and organs

- *Majja* ( marrow), manufacturing blood and the adjacent nervous system running through the hollows of the bones sending and receiving messages from the brain
- *Shukra* (reproductive tissue), the sexual organ systems creating and sustaining the life force

When the essential energy of the immune system(or *Ojas,* meaning "vigor" in Sanskrit), becomes weakened through years of dietary abuse, poor digestion, stress and trauma, toxins accumulate to a point were they overflow and search for weak areas in the body to locate, eventually manifesting as full blown disease symptoms such as pain and inflammation.

It is at this stage that most cancers are diagnosed. It has usually been accumulating in the body for a period of time. It is different in each circumstance, but a series of factors involving poor diet, emotional stress, environmental pollution, genetics and inharmonious personal relationships, all combine to create an immune deficiency causing the cells of the body to malfunction. It doesn't matter where in the body the cancer shows up, in the tissues or an organ, a muscle, the blood, the brain, the reproductive system, etc, this only provides a label for it. This is the area in the body that was the most vulnerable to attack and that is where the symptom will manifest.

The qualities of the *doshas* - cold and dryness for *Vata*, heat and inflammation for *Pitta* and damp and congestion for *Kapha* - become vitiated or unstable. Then they enter the *dhatus* (tissues) and start to cause trouble in the following ways:

## The Six Stages of Disease

Ayurveda explains how disease progresses by stages if the early warning signs are not recognized and treated. The qualities of the *doshas* increase because of aggravating factors such as stress and wrong diet, change of climate, emotional upheaval etc. These factors weaken the digestive fire which in turn creates undigested toxins (*ama*), that stick in the micro channels (*srotas*), the body's bio-transport system. This causes blockages and overflows, thereby obstructing the flow of essential nutrients, causing deficiencies in the body.

If each stage is unaddressed, the symptoms become more aggressive and proceed to the next stage. Eventually they accumulate in the weakest area of the body in the form of undifferentiated cancer cells which form tumors and attack the organs.

## The Six Stages

1. Accumulation : toxins build up

2. Aggravation : they become inflamed

3. Overflow or Spread : they start to move

4. Localization : they find a weak spot to attack

5. Manifestation : specific physical symptoms appear

6. Diversification : chronic complications ensue

If caught in the first three stages, the disease is easier to treat. Once it moves to a weak area of the body and settles in, the disease has had time to gain strength and it is more difficult to treat. It requires a more rigorous intervention to turn it around and the treatment and recovery period is much longer.

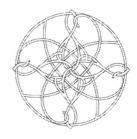

# CHAPTER 37

# *AGNI*

## (THE DIGESTIVE FIRE)

*" He who worships agni, will be blessed with perfect health "*
Dr Vasant Lad

EVERYONE is familiar with the saying "You are what you eat" but that's only partially true because more specifically, "You are what you digest!" It is said in Ayurveda that every disease can be traced to poor digestion. When you think about it, your body is the product of trillions of cells constantly being created to support some form of tissue in the body. These cells are constantly multiplying and dividing to form the skin, bones, muscles, nails, hair and the various organs.

The nutrients to feed and grow these cells efficiently come from the food we eat, the liquid we drink and the air we breathe. On a quantum level the cells are also fed by the perceptual images and emotional states of the conscious and sub-conscious mind. If our digestive system is not assimilating and metabolizing these nutrients efficiently, some part of the body will be under-nourished, the immune system will be compromised and disease may result.

The Sanskrit word *agni* refers to the biological digestive fire of transformation and transmutation. The primary function of *agni* is the digestion, assimilation and absorption of food, emotions and sensations. If one is not hungry and eats anyway, or eats too much junk food, or eats too fast or when emotionally upset, the food will not be broken down efficiently by the various acids and enzymes in the stomach. The bulky, undigested particles (**ama**), become sticky and instead of being evacuated by the bowels, can get stuck in the intestinal walls, eventually leaching into the body accumulating as toxins that clog the system. This can result in constipation, or, alternatively, the body may reject the food entirely, forcing it though the system to be released as diarrhea. You put junk in, you get junk out!

It is all the more important then to keep our digestive systems happy. This can be achieved not only by eating the right seasonal fresh foods for our body type, but by also eating at the right time of day. Breakfast should be taken between 7-8 am. Lunch should be the main meal of the day and eaten when the sun is at its zenith around 12-1 pm. This is *pitta* time when our appetite is strongest and this food becomes the fuel for the activity to come in the rest of the day. The evening meal should be light and easy to digest at around 6-7 pm, at least 2 to 3 hours before bed. This is *kapha* time and is for rest and relaxation after the activities of the day and to give time for the food to be digested before sleeping. Intervals of 4 to 5 hours between meals is best, without snacking and grazing in between which, as your Mother told you, will spoil your appetite. If your digestive system is working properly, you will not feel hunger between meals.

# Guidelines for Eating

## Mindfulness

Our salivation starts when we think of food. Our sense organs can often pressure us into making good or bad choices. How then should we approach the eating of food with a conscious understanding of what is best for us? We rush around so much during the day that we don't take the time to sit and eat properly. When we talk about mindful eating we imagine a monk, eating a simple bowl of rice with no thought of doing anything else but eating. He is not talking or reading the paper or watching TV. He is just eating. There are so many distractions around us in today's world, it takes some practice to enjoy this simple act. When we eat consciously, our digestive system works optimally.

Eat in a peaceful clean environment. Eating food that is lightly cooked is easier on the digestion. Eat organic, locally grown, seasonal foods that your body will adapt to more easily. Before eating say a prayer of thanks asking for nourishment for the body. Your attitude about the food you eat is important. In time your body will come to know intuitively if a food is good for you and you will make decisions based on your best interests. Stop eating before you feel full. Leave a little feeling of hunger and in 10 minutes of sitting quietly you will feel quite satisfied. This is the way to prevent over eating and indigestion.

Cooking is a skill that can be taught. When you love to cook for yourself or others, you will impart that love into the food and it will be more nutritious and digestible. Avoid frozen food or food that is heated in a microwave. The molecular structure of the food has been altered negatively by these actions. Forget about everything when eating. Eat outside or gaze out of a window at nature if possible. You will be amazed at how well your digestion works when you do this. Try not to eat when you are feeling negative emotions or when you are not hungry.

Here are some guidelines for consciously eating and digesting food:

- Always take time to eat quietly and slowly
- Chew food thoroughly before swallowing
- Never eat if you are emotionally upset
- Eat fresh, lightly cooked food
- Do not speak when chewing

- Sip a cup of hot water for easier digestion
- Eat with good company if possible
- Stop eating when three-quarters full
- Sit quietly for a few minutes after your meal

Sounds simple doesn't it? If you practice this you will digest and assimilate your food better in the manner we call **sattvic** or balanced. This naturally leads to greater health. Try it and see for yourself how much happier it will make you feel after every meal.

## The Six Tastes

Each meal should contain the six tastes whenever possible. In India special attention is given to this practice. It helps to stimulate different aspects of the digestive process by releasing different enzymes to assist in absorption of the food. Here are the six tastes and some examples of food that contain them:

- Sweet        sugar, rice, wheat, milk, dates
- Sour         lemon, lime, grapefruit, pickles, yogurt
- Salty        sea salt, seaweed, celery, avocado
- Pungent      cayenne, chilies, pepper, garlic, ginger, onion
- Bitter       lentils, dandelion, artichoke, turmeric, coffee
- Astringent   leafy greens, green tea, cardamom, pomegranate, apples

Small amounts of these tastes are contained in many cooking spices and they add flavor as well as digestive aid. A good way to stimulate the appetite is to slice a thin wedge of ginger about the size of a quarter and add a little celtic salt and a squeeze of lime or lemon. Chew and swallow before meals.

The restaurant obsession with providing a large glass of iced water could not be more counter-productive. The cold water drowns the digestive fire. Better to sip hot water during meals to help kindle the fire and break down the food particles.

In today's working world it is often not possible to eat a good, hot meal in the middle of the day, but don't be tempted to skip this meal. Take a wide mouth thermos filled with a hot protein rich food to eat on your lunch break. Probably one of the most effective things we can do to keep our appetites sharp, is to eat at regular times each day. This way we train our appetite and the digestive fire *(agni)* to peak so that we are able to maximize the assimilation of the valuable nutrients in our food.

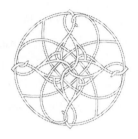

# CHAPTER 38

# THE AYURVEDA LIFE

*"Two hours sleep before midnight is worth four hours after midnight"*
Old Japanese Saying

## A GOOD NIGHT'S SLEEP

EVERYDAY the environment is ecologically bombarding our senses and mind, causing stress and disease. What we feel and perceive in our mind and bodies takes a toll on our system and our batteries get run down. If we do not take time to recharge them we eventually collapse. The body has its own natural way of recharging itself through our sleeping hours, but we often do not acknowledge this natural healing pattern that is available to us every night.

There is a saying that goes, "Two hours of sleep before midnight is worth four hours after midnight." This means that getting to bed by 10 pm is one of the healthiest things you can do for your body, *especially* if you are recovering from an illness. The period between 10pm and 2am is when the deepest, most rejuvenating sleep occurs. In the two hours between 10 and 12 pm, the natural hormone melatonin is released into the brain to provide deep sleep. It is the time when the body goes into its automatic repair mode to recover from the activities of the previous day.

This is the 4 hour period when the liver and spleen are processing blood and removing the daily accumulation of toxic material, sending it to the kidneys and excretory glands for expulsion from the body. This is why you wake to pee in the night and evacuate the bowels first thing in the morning. The heart and lungs slow their rhythms and gentle re-oxygenation of millions of cells takes place.

Of all the resources available to us to heal the body, sleep is the most important to recognize. It takes no effort and it's free! If you are a "night owl" and have trouble getting to bed early, try getting up between 6 and 7am for 3 mornings in a row. This will begin to make you tired at night and train your body to desire an earlier bedtime. On the fourth day put the lights out at 10pm and you will begin to retrain yourself to get 8 hours of sleep in harmony with the natural setting and rising of the sun.

This is your natural biological rhythm, and by habituating yourself to staying up late to "get more work done" you are setting the stage for imbalance and illness, be it a stress related common cold or something more chronic, accumulated over time. Don't take naps during the day, this is like spoiling your appetite by snacking between meals; you will not create the natural tiredness that is needed for a good nights sleep.

If you are recovering from cancer this early 8 hour pattern is especially important. In fact in this case, *it is crucial to allow the body to sleep whenever it wants*, and naps are a good thing. The body must work overtime to do the processing needed to repair the cells and eliminate the unwanted detritus that is left over from the effects of chemotherapy and/or radiation. If your sleep patterns are disturbed because of illness, stress, or anxiety, try taking Melatonin, a natural hormone, available at your local natural food store. Experiment with the dose that is right for you. Here is an Ayurvedic herbal formula for helping nightly sleep.

Boil a glass of raw or whole organic milk until it froths. Remove from heat and add

- 1 tsp Ashwagandha powder,
- 1 pinch turmeric powder
- 1 pinch cinnamon
- 1 pinch cardamom
- 1 pinch nutmeg
- ¼ tsp raw honey.

Drink this warm right before bed. If you cannot get the Ashwagandha from your health food store, the other combination of ingredients works fine too. You may also dilute the milk with ½ cup of water. Sweet dreams.

## How to Begin the Day

How you begin the night will determine how you begin your day.

If you go to sleep early you will wake early. You will wake refreshed and eager to greet the new day's challenges. If you have cancer or are dealing with any form of illness, you are giving yourself a head start by getting enough restful sleep. When you begin to recover you will have many more good days than bad and you will be able to perform the daily routines with energy and enthusiasm.

It's preferable to wake up before the sun. This is a quiet time of meditative calm. You may choose to review dreams or write in a journal but it is usually best to begin a meditative period first while everything is still peaceful. Sit in a relaxed position on a pillow or in a chair. You may begin by doing breathing exercises and follow with meditation or reverse it or combine them both.

Do some light yoga stretches combined with deep breathing for a few minutes to wake the body up. Next begin the cleaning regimen. Oil the body with a light self massage from head to toe. This is called *Abhyanga* in Ayurveda and you can use sesame or coconut oil. It takes about 5 minutes for a light rub all over the body including the head and hair if you intend to wash it that day. Try to leave the oil on the body for 5 to 15 minutes, or as long as possible prior to bathing, this will help the skin to absorb it.

Scrape the tongue and brush and floss the teeth, then do what is called '*Neti*', pouring warm salt water through the nostrils to clear the sinuses and improve breathing. There is a special little pot called a *neti* pot available for this, with instructions at most health food stores. This is not as strange as it may sound and as a daily practice will prevent colds and flu, clear the sinuses and free up your breathing.

Now the hot shower, which will help the oil penetrate the tissues, followed by a cold rinse to bring the blood to the surface. If you have a bath, or better still a hot tub, you may want to soak to allow the muscles to relax. After drying off, follow with a dry brush massage to stimulate the lymph and remove any unwanted dead skin from the surface pores.

At some stage you may want to introduce a little more exercise such as walking, rebounding, Qi gong or yoga. Depending on what my body feels like that day, I like to do my exercise at this time to stimulate my appetite before breakfast. To do all this, from the time of waking up to breakfast, can take any where from 1 to 2 hours depending on your energy level and health goals, but I assure you when it becomes a daily routine it will make a big difference to your health. You may find friends commenting that you look like you're glowing and they will want to know what your secret to radiant health is. This is a reward in itself.

Of course this is an ideal day and in a recovery from illness, or during rough patches, you may only do part or none of this. You have to feel into your body each morning and decide what is best for you that day. It is better to do nothing rather than force something and feel worse. There is an Ayurvedic phrase for this called '*pravabha paradha*' which translated means "A crime of the intellect", in other words, doing something you know is not good for you. So be gentle with yourself and start slowly. Build up to a daily practice that serves you best in the moment of choice.

# MEDITATION, YOGA AND PRANAYAMA

One of the main differences between Ayurveda and its Western allopathic counterpart, is the way Ayurveda always approaches the well being of a person from a holistic point of view, with the idea of first *removing the cause* of any disease. The four essential aspects of the human being are viewed as Body, Mind, Senses and Soul (or Consciousness). There is no healing without addressing all of these aspects.

Conversely, to take the Western point of view toward treatment, the thinking is always scientific and sees the health of a person as the absence of disease. It tries to tackle disease by isolating, palliating or eradicating the symptoms. Rather than looking at the whole person, it is reductionist and mechanistic. It is based on the Descartes view of the body as a machine which can be fixed by mending the broken part.

The health of any human being must be looked at from an enlightened, loving perspective. Ayurvedic practitioners are encouraged to *"fall in love"* with their patients first, otherwise healing is not possible. Is the person whole, happy and emotionally balanced? In Sanskrit the word for this balanced state is *satwic,* which means full of clarity, vitally aware and harmoniously in tune with nature. We should settle for nothing less.

It is not just by right diet, proper sleep and a good exercise program that this profound state is achieved. The practice of daily meditation has a highly beneficial effect on health and especially the recovery from illness. Add to this the exercise of gentle stretching called yoga and a conscious breathing practice called pranayama, and you have a powerful, threefold recipe for healing and long life.

## Meditation

Everyone is familiar with meditation. Its benefits include increased mental acuity, clarity, insight and awareness. As a stress reducer it is unparalleled. If you are a newcomer to mediation, just 10 minutes a day will begin to have an effect over time. Sit in a quiet place where you will not be disturbed by anyone. Close your eyes and allow thoughts and images to arise and, as much as possible, do not get pulled into their content. Instead, focus on your breathing and watch the breath flow in and out through the nostrils. Fill the belly and the chest, and let it flow out again with no effort to control it. Over time your ability to come to a neutral place, where thoughts continue but are not consciously observed, will improve with practice and longer periods of sitting will become natural. Always try to set aside the same time everyday, whether it is morning or evening or both, so that it becomes a regular habit.

## Yoga

Gentle stretching combined with the breath is a powerful healing exercise. It has been practiced in the East for hundreds of years in many different forms. Hatha Yoga, with its many variations, is now main-stream in the US and you can find a group practice on any given day in most towns. Even doing a simple Sun Salutation, a series of 6 or 7 moves in a specific sequence, every morning after arising, or in the evening after work, will benefit breathing, posture and blood flow. Take a class, buy a book or watch a DVD and become familiar with this ancient exercise. Just the regular practice of laying on your back on the floor for 10 minutes when you return from a days work, will allow the body to begin its healing from the stressful activities of the day. By doing this you will allow your body to 'catch up' with itself and you will get up feeling rejuvenated.

# The Headstand

Once you become more adept at Yoga, and particularly for those with cancer or recovering from it, the following instructions will help you learn a very powerful healing practice. This may seem a little esoteric if you are not familiar with it, but I assure you that with practice it is not difficult to do and it will increase your healing capacity, improve your mental clarity and, as the famous Yogi B.S Ayengar stated when he did a headstand on the edge of the Grand Canyon, "If you do this for 10 minutes a day, it will add 10 years to your life"

This is called a triangle headstand. Find a wall and kneel down facing it preferably on a cushioned surface. Interlock your fingers and place your hands just behind and on top of your head. Now bend forward and place the top of your head on the floor about 8 inches away from the wall. Keep your elbows about 18 inches apart. The backs of your hands and forearms should form a triangle cradling your head. These will take the majority of the weight of your body. Now lift up your knees, straighten your legs and walk slowly towards the wall. When you have formed an inverted 'vee' with your body, kick your legs up against the wall supporting your weight on your forearms. Some weight will bear down onto the top of your head but you should be able to take the majority onto your clasped hands and arms.

Begin with short periods until your arms gain strength and when you get tired come back down slowly by bending your knees and tipping your weight back onto your feet. With practice you will be able to maintain longer periods and eventually become comfortable without the wall for support. Three to five minutes a day will accelerate any healing process and encourage blood flow and lymph drainage.

Caution: Do not practice this if you have a history of heart problems, osteoporosis or are unfamiliar with simple Yoga postures. Substitute a simple modified shoulder stand and get the same benefits of an inverted posture. One can even sit next to a wall on the left side, then swing the body at right angles to the wall while laying down and rest the legs up against the wall. Just doing this simple pose for five minutes a day is extremely restorative for the body.

## Pranayama

There are many and varied breathing techniques all lumped under the word Pranayama. Any of these is an added benefit to exercise and only requires you to sit in a comfortable position with a straight back.

Here is a description of one exercise, using alternate nostril breathing, called **nadishodhana** in Sanskrit. It will clear the mind, refresh the lungs and nasal passages, and at the same time generate the life force energy called Prana.

## Alternate Nostril Breathing *(Nadishodhana)*

Close your right nostril with the thumb of your right hand. Breathe in slowly and deeply through your left nostril for a count of 5. Now also cover your left nostril with the ring finger (next to the pinky) of your right hand and hold both nostrils for a count of 5. Open you right nostril and breathe out for a count of 10. Still keeping the left nostril closed breathe in through the right nostril for another count of 5. Close both nostrils again for the count of 5. Open the left nostril and breathe out for a count of 10. Repeat this sequence for about 5 minutes. If you feel dizzy shorten the breath counts to what feels comfortable and avoid holding the breath in the middle. Do this before or after meditation for maximum effect.

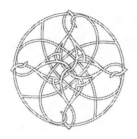

# CHAPTER 39

# *PANCHA KARMA*
# CLEANSING THE BODY

*"No disease will go unless the root is cut.*
*When disease has already set in,*
*it will not go unless the body is purified."*

Dr. R.H.Singh, B.A.M.S

**P**ANCHA Karma literally means 'Five Actions'. It is a group of integrated treatments designed to flush out toxins, replenish nutrients and rejuvenate the whole body/mind. It is normally recommended that a person do at least some of these procedures every year in the Spring and Fall to cleanse the body and prevent disease from forming.

Everyone picks up some form of toxins everyday, whether it is from the chemicals in our food or from environmental pollution. Further toxins build up in our system because of poor digestion. In the case of more serious disease such as cancer, that has reached a critical point in its development, it becomes necessary to flush the body of these impurities, cleanse the blood, and rejuvenate the immune system to effect any sort of healing.

Kerala State, in the South West corner of India, has some of the most authentic clinics practicing this ancient art of healing. The SNA Ayurvedic Nursing Home in Thrissur, that I have attended on several occasions, has documents dating back over 1,000 years of Ayurvedic practicing history. This medical knowledge has been handed down through 18 generations to the present day.

The current clinic, founded in 1920 by the Mooss family joined forces with the Nambi family. The Chief Physician, *Ashtavaidyan* Alathiyoor Narayanan Nambi, a Master Practitioner, now in his 70's, still practices everyday alongside his daughter-in law, the lovely Dr. Devi Narayanan. The new 15 room clinic is overseen by Deputy Chief Physician and Managing Director, *Ashtavaidyan* PTN Vasudevan Mooss. SNA also have their own herbal factory producing all their medicinal formulas. You can view their website at www.moossayurveda.com or email at www.drmoos@gmail.com

In 2010 they opened a new facility in the large town of Thrissur, about an hours taxi ride from Kochi Airport. The 15 room clinic is in a relatively quiet area within 15 minutes walk of the town's center circle, a one way traffic system around an enormous ancient Hindu temple and elephant sanctuary.

The accommodations in the clinic are simple and clean. The food is vegetarian, tasty and always served on time. The large staff are friendly and skillful and the weekly cost is very inexpensive. The quality of care is first class and the treatments are traditional, authentic and the best you will find anywhere in India.

If you go to Kerala for *pancha karma* treatment, plan on being there for a month if possible. The treatments are given every morning and afternoon and run in 7 day cycles, so allowing 28 days is best. This will give you time to acclimatize to the moist, humid weather. October, November is the coolest time of year when the warm, southwest monsoons cool the air and make the tropical vegetation come alive. Bring light clothing, a good novel and an open mind, and you will fall in love with Kerala and her people.

Here are the "five actions" or treatments of traditional *Keraliya pancha karma*. Each one has dozens of variations based on your specific health concerns, your particular constitution, and the hundreds of medicinal herbs and oils available to treat the body.

### *Kaya Seca or Pizhichil* (*Piri-chil*)

The body is flooded with hot herbal infused oil poured from silver pots by four therapists, two on each side, and massaged into the body with long, sweeping, rhythmical strokes. The massage table is called a ***dhoni,*** often carved from a solid block of wood. The oil is channeled to a drain in the end of the table where it is collected by a fifth person, reheated and reapplied to the body.

Just as a stick will become more flexible if first soaked in water, so the body softens as it takes in the oil and the herbs via trans-dermal feeding of the muscles and tissues beneath the skin. This forces the body to release toxins via the perspiration. It is used for rejuvenation, healthy ageing, and all neurological and nervous disorders such as Parkinson's, paraplegia, M.S. and other chronic diseases.

### *Navarakizhi (Nava-ra-kiri)*

A nutritious type of rice called Navara is cooked in a decoction of herbs and milk. The boiled rice is then strained, wrapped in linen cloths and tied with a knot. The cloth ball of rice is the size of a softball and called a bolus. First the body is massaged with warm oil and then the cloth bolus' are heated in the hot milk. Two people apply the hot bolus' to the body's front, back and two sides by massaging them into the skin. A thick, white slurry paste from the rice is built up covering the whole body and this is massaged into the skin. It is eventually removed with the soft edge of coconut palm leaves. Finally a hot bath is taken by pouring water over yourself from a large plastic tub. Then, as with all these treatments, an hour of rest is prescribed.

This treatment is used for all conditions. It provides muscle power, skin rejuvenation and detoxification. It is used specifically for arthritis and neurological disorders.

### Shirodhara (Sheero-dara)

**Shiro** is head and **dhara** means flow. After a warm oil massage the person lays on their back with the head cushioned at the end of the table. A warm flow of herbal infused oil or milk flows over the forehead and the top of the skull from a bowl suspended above the head. In Ayurveda the top of the head is likened to the roots of a tree because this is where the herbal nutrients can best be absorbed by the nervous system of the body.

This procedure stimulates a micro vibration in the skull, synchronizing the nervous system and producing a muscular relaxation response. It is excellent for multiple conditions to feed and rejuvenate the body and relieve stress.

### Udvartana (ood-var-tana)

This type of massage uses a cereal paste made from the flours of bran and lentils, coconut, sesame and herbs. It is mixed with oil, yogurt and honey to produce a "chocolate pudding" paste. After massaging the body with warm oil, the paste is rubbed into the skin in a flowing motion by two people (always men with men and women with women), working in harmony, with identical strokes, either side of the patient. The paste begins to dry, cooling the body, drawing out toxins and at the same time supplying nutrients to the skin. Coconut palm fronds are used to scrape off the paste before a warm bath and rest.

### Basti (vasti)

This is an enema using medicated oil formulas or milk and ghee, often containing combinations of medicinal herbs. It is the most powerful of the Kerala treatments and there are over 50 different formulas for specific conditions. It helps dispel disease rapidly from the body with its flushing effect and also adds nutrients and healing herbs by absorption through the walls of the intestines. It is a powerful detoxification agent and helps to rejuvenate the body by flushing out unwanted matter and cleansing the whole system. It rejuvenates, provides strength and long life, and improves the overall complexion. It can enrich the bacterial flora of the intestinal walls and affects the neurological functions of the brain and nervous system.

These are the main *pancha karma* treatments of the Kerala region although there are many variations and each clinic will have its own traditional style. The Kerala treatments differ from the 'Classical' style of Northern India in that they are less invasive and geared more toward balancing and rejuvenation.

Many of these treatments are available in some form at Ayurveda centers in the United States, although because of labor costs, there will rarely be more than two therapists in attendance. Treatment periods are shorter, mainly because of the cost factor, but they are still very effective in treating disease, recovery from illness or for cleansing and rejuvenation. Cost of treatment varies depending on the "Spa" factor and number of therapists involved, but can range anywhere from $200 to $500 per day.

The cost of a month's treatment in Kerala is usually around $300 a week for everything. This includes two treatments a day, several specially formulated herbal medicines a day (including two months post treatment supply to take home), and all food and accommodation. Even adding in the airfare it is still a fraction of the cost of treatment in the U.S. The only downside is the long journey but, if you are well enough to travel, I highly advise giving yourself the real deal. When you return, be sure to allow several weeks to re-integrate, allowing time for the treatments to sink in. You will usually feel the benefits in the following months as the body adapts to the cleansing.

If you don't want to travel that far, then try a shorter version in the U.S. There are now, increasingly more, very good Ayurvedic Treatment Centers available in many states. I can recommend the following: Dr. John Doulliard in Boulder, Colorado,www.lifespar.com.

Shekhar Annaambhotla in Coopersburg, Pennsylvania, www.ojas.us.

Ambika Copple at the Lotus in Santa Cruz, California, and Deanna Batdorff's 'Dhyana Center of Health Sciences' in Sebastopol, California. www.info@ dhyanacenter.com

## Summary of Ayurvedic Principles

We started with the *doshas,,* the collective term for the three biological modes or constitutional types, determined at birth by your genetic make-up. They are *vata,* movement, change and wind, having the elements of air and ether. Next is *pitta,* all about focus, transformation and digestion, having the elements of fire and water and lastly *kapha*, compassion, stability and cohesion having the elements of earth and water. When the *doshas* are stressed by calamity, and become unbalanced, they attack the *dhatus* (tissues) and cause disease.

There are 7 *dhatus* or tissue layers comprising of plasma, blood, muscle, fat, bone, marrow and reproductive tissue. When the body is healthy and *agni,* (the biological fire of digestion and transformation), is strong, the immune system, *(ojas),* supports the *dhatus,* and prevents them from becoming weak and susceptible to disease.

Through physical and emotional stress, unsuitable lifestyle choices, environmental toxins, poor diet, etc, the body becomes unable to properly digest the food we eat. Over time toxins *(ama),* build up in the body causing illness and disease. So it is by living conscious, healthy lifestyles and eating a diet that is current with the seasons and correctly suited for our type, getting proper exercise, using breath and meditation and doing regular cleansing *(pancha karma),* that we can optimize our health and prevent disease.

Study the following charts to determine what constitutional type (*dosha*) you are and see what foods best suit you. These are not meant as rigid rules. In Ayurveda it is said, "Everything depends...." Depends on what you might ask? Depends on what your constitution is, the state of your health, your age, where in the world you live, what season it is, what time of day it is, what food grows locally, etc. Because each of us is a unique combination of all three *doshas*, each of our needs can change from day to day, and even moment to moment. As we become more aware of our bodies, and how to live in harmony with the natural rhythms of life, we become healthier and more vital.

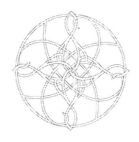

# CHAPTER 40

# *DOSHA* SELF-EVALUATION CHARTS

## PHYSICAL AND EMOTIONAL CHARACTERISTICS

### *VATA* : (Change)

| | |
|---|---|
| Elements | Ether and Air |
| Body Type | Light, thin, boney or wiry body frame with prominent veins. Taller or shorter than average. Difficulty gaining weight and usually underweight. Thin wrists and bone structure. Long fingers. |
| Features | Curly, kinky or fine hair. Rough or dry skin with cracking nails and joints. Cold hands and feet with aversion to cold damp or windy weather. Speech is fast and talkative, sometimes missing words. |
| Digestion | Variable. Often skips meals or lack of interest in eating. |

Tendency to constipation, bloating and gas.

| | |
|---|---|
| Energy | Swings from high to low. Can become fatigued from over-exertion. Often has multiple projects happening and have difficulty with completion. Can "crash and burn" from over-doing. Light sleeper, suffers from insomnia. |
| Emotions | Tendency toward anxiety, fear and doubt. Sometimes over-analyze and plan excessively before taking action. Can also act impulsively. Sometimes overly sensitive nature and when hurt will cry. Expresses emotions with words and likes to talk a lot. Learns things quickly but forgets immediately. |
| General Qualities | Money "runs through their fingers". Likes travel, exercise, change and variety in life. Uncomfortable when still. Creative, artistic people leading to careers in the Arts or service providers. Can see the 'big picture' but lack focus making decisions. |
| Animal Characteristic | Deer, rabbit |

## PITTA: (Focus)

| | |
|---|---|
| Elements | Fire and Water |
| Body Type | Medium build, athletic. Physically strong and active, they tend to act quickly and to "shoot first and ask questions later." |

| | |
|---|---|
| Features | Often have a reddish, flushed complexion with sharp nose, tongue and teeth. Reddish/auburn or soft brown hair with receding hairline and early balding. Fair, shiny skin and bright eyes. Heart shaped face with freckles or moles. Do not tolerate heat and bright sunlight. Speech is sharp and clear cut. |
| Digestion | Strong digestive fire with tendency to eat fast and not chew food properly. Large capacity to eat and assimilate large variety of food.. Becomes irritable if they miss meals. Difficulty with hot, spicy food. Able to tolerate more raw foods and a variety of animal products. When imbalanced can experience diarrhea or soft stools. When the urge comes to defecate, they "have to go" immediately. |
| Energy | Strong active fire with competitive nature leading to burn-out and over heating. Can be fun people making good leaders with the ability to focus and complete tasks. |
| Emotions | Tendency toward anger, jealousy and hate. Can be sharp and cutting in conversation. Tendency toward perfection and control. |
| General Qualities | Don't like change much and like to have a stable place to call home which is generally orderly and neat. A good organizer, likes to be an entrepreneur, CEO or Lawyer. Can |

save money but a big spender. Sharp, intelligent and analytical, they make good leaders. When challenged they will argue and fight. They express their emotions with gifts.

| | |
|---|---|
| Animal | Tiger, Lion |

# KAPHA: (Nourishment)

| | |
|---|---|
| Elements | Water and Earth |
| Body Type | Large body frame with heavy bones and muscles, tendency to gain and hold weight. Grounded, stable and slow moving. Weight and holding water can lead to congestion, sluggishness and an aversion to exercise. |
| Features | Often has thick, lustrous hair, large eyes with clear sclera, straight even teeth, pale color and soft, oily, moist, thick skin. Large features with round face. Ages well and often looks younger. Speech is slow, clear and sweet. |
| Digestion | Steady appetite and regular elimination. Able to eat a variety of foods but does best with lighter more raw diet. Often skips breakfast and has large lunch. Likes sweet things but does best when avoiding dairy, breads and mucous producing food. |
| Energy | Slow moving but with good endurance and strength. Can be lethargic but with great |

stamina once they get going. Often desires coffee as a stimulant in the morning. Tendency to stay up late and likes to sleep in. Generally maintain good health with few illnesses.

Emotions

Compassionate, kind and forgiving. Loves to hug and communicates through touch. Can become attached to people and things leading to avarice and procrastination. Strong humanitarian, mothering and nurturing influence and sensitive to others feelings. Moods are steady and unchanging.

General Qualities

Usually a soft, big hearted person who likes to socialize and care for others but tends not to nourish themselves. You will always get a great hug from a kapha person. They like regularity and are slow and deliberate in action, disliking last minute changes to their carefully laid plans. They are slow to learn but can retain information and have a good memory. They are thoughtful, compassionate human beings often in the care giving professions. When challenged they will withdraw or try to make peace. They are good savers and accumulate wealth.

Animal

Bear, Swan, Elephant.

# *DOSHA*
# FOOD PREFERENCE CHARTS

This is only a general outline, as individual circumstances involving age, season, general state of health and the stage of any cancer has to be a factor in determining an appropriate diet. All three *doshas* should cook their green leafy vegetables slightly. This will not destroy any significant amount of their potency and will make them more digestible. All types should favor the brassica varieties (i.e. cabbage, broccoli and cauliflower), which are known to prevent cancer.

These charts were compiled with the help of Dr. Vasant Lad and Usha Lad's excellent book, "Ayurvedic Cooking for Self-Healing".

## VATA

The *Vata* individual, with a cold, dry constitution usually does better with a diet of warm, soupy foods. Their healthy tastes are sweet, salty and sour. Soups, casseroles, stews, warm fruit desserts and hot herbal teas, all suit *Vata* no matter the season. They have a high metabolism so three good meals a day is best with the possible need to supplement with a protein snack to prevent hypoglycemia as long as their appetite is not compromised. They can be so busy they forget about eating regularly and food is not the first thing on their mind come lunchtime. *Vata* does well on a good solid breakfast whether it be hot oatmeal or an omelet. Their dry, light nature is not conducive to chips, popcorn or dried grains like muesli and granola.

They should favor cooked vegetables over raw and eat mostly sweet fruits and dried fruits in moderation. They do not digest soy well except in its fermented state such as miso and tempeh. Nuts and seeds are good and they can usually tolerate dairy and some meat protein. Best oils are sesame, olive and ghee. Supplements should include bee pollen, royal jelly, and blue-green algae. Minerals are calcium, copper, iron, magnesium and zinc. Vitamins, A, all B's, C, D, E and Folic Acid.

## PITTA

Pitta individuals are the great transformers and they often have the ability to consume large amounts of food in a short time with a strong digestive power. If they are late eating their appetite will 'fire' up and make them irritable and unusually unfocused until they can balance themselves by re-fueling. Because of their fiery nature they do not necessarily do well with fried or spicy dishes and are more suited to cooling, raw foods and white meats and freshwater fish.

Pitta's best tastes are sweet and bitter and they should favor vegetables like cilantro, cooked leafy greens, salads, celery and eat mostly sweet fruit. They can digest most beans including soy and the fermented products. Dairy is usually tolerated in moderation, but nuts can be aggravating. It is best to use coconut milk with its oil and meat. Avoiding excessive use of stimulants like alcohol and caffeine and using cool fruit drinks and herbal teas will help to keep them balanced.

Supplement with Aloe Vera, Barley Green and Brewers Yeast. Add minerals calcium, magnesium zinc. Use spirulina and blue green-algae along with vitamins A, B1, B12, D and K.

## KAPHA

Kapha types are able to eat a wide variety of food and digest it well with one or two notable exceptions. Because of their wet and cool constitution they do not do well with dairy. Milk and cheeses cause them congestion, as does wheat and baked goodies, which they tend to love. Their tendency to gain weight at the mere sight of bread makes them better suited to a more raw and vegetarian diet. Drier grains work better for them such as cold cereals like muesli and granola, millet and quinoa.

Their tastes are pungent and bitter and they can handle more spicy foods. They should favor these kinds of vegetables, kale, leeks, daikon radish, burdock and dandelion greens. Because of their sweet tooth, Kapha should avoid sweet fruits and go for astringent apples, pears and berries. Unfortunately nuts are-not good but they can use flax, chia, hemp, sunflower and pumpkin seeds.

Kapha people tend to move more slowly and like their morning sleep; for this reason they will have enough reserves to skip breakfast and make lunch their first food of the day. Baked and grilled vegetables and meats are easier on their system. All spices are good but they should go easy on the salt. Small amounts of sunflower or sesame oil and ghee are good for cooking with.

Mineral supplements should include copper, iron. Calcium, magnesium and zinc, blue green-algae and the vitamins B6, C and folic acid.

# EPILOGUE

## Finding *Your* Way

*"There is a small space within the heart that contains everything.*
*In the infinitesimal we can find the infinite.*
*What we call the mind is a deeper awareness of the heart as*
*a manifestation of everything, everywhere; an awareness*
*that is beyond the senses We are all stimulated and depressed.*
*We live in the outer world and need to learn*
*to move into the inner world at the core of our Being which*
*is the Being that is everywhere.*
*Seeing, hearing and speaking this unity*
*which is at the core of the heart,*
*is the essence of healing"*

David Frawley
Speaking at the 2010 NAMA
Conference Panel in San Francisco

I eventually found my way to health again after searching many avenues. Some were dead ends, but most offered a way out of my predicament. I had to find *my* own way. Now you must find yours.

Your way will be unique to you and your needs. Be inquisitive and determined in your search. Don't give up if you hit a wall. Turn around and start again. Be persistent and listen to your body. It knows how to heal itself and you will be guided to choose the right path.

Work with your health-care providers and physicians but only if they will work with you. You are in charge of your healing process and you have to make the final decisions about the roads you want to travel down, be it an Integrative approach along side western medicine, or a completely natural, alternative one, choosing the healing methods you are drawn to. Your body will let you know. Slow down and get used to listening to it.

There are no guarantees during this lifetime. This place is a school and it is all a grand experiment to learn to love and be loved while we are alive. We will pass on some time and our Spirit will rejoice in the next adventure. Ultimately, we don't know what will happen next, but I believe we all have invisible guides or passed over loved ones, call them Angels if you like, that are always with us in every moment. We can call upon them at any time. My experience is that when we are stuck, or in a difficult place, they will do what it takes to show us the way forward - *if we ask them and if we listen*. Meditation, dreams and prayer are our allies in this life, be sure to use them.

In my opinion there are three little words that are very wonderful to say and to hear in our lives and they're not what you might think. These words are "I AM WELL!" When someone next asks how we are and we can say those three words confidently in reply, this is a privilege we take all too often for granted. Think about it. We can have wealth, possessions, status, and even love, but if we don't have health, it is difficult to appreciate and enjoy any of these things. However, if we have health, all of the above will come with it automatically. When illness strikes and our very life is threatened, that's when our health becomes precious. When you earn the right to say "I AM WELL!" you will never take life for granted again. I hope this book will put you and your loved ones on that road to wellness

EPILOGUE

May You Be Well.
May You Be Happy,
May All Beings Be at Peace

*Happiness cannot be found*
*through great effort and willpower,*
*but is already present, in open relaxation and letting go.*
*Don't strain yourself,*
*there is nothing to do or undo.*
*Whatever momentarily arises in the body-mind*
*has no real importance at all,*
*has little reality whatsoever.*
*Why identify with, and become attached to it,*
*passing judgment upon it and ourselves?*
*Far better to simply*
*let the entire game happen on its own,*
*springing up and falling back like waves -*
*without changing or manipulating anything -*
*and notice how every thing vanishes and*
*reappears, magically, again and again,*
*time without end.*
*Only our searching for happiness*
*prevents us from seeing it.*
*It's like a vivid rainbow which you pursue without ever catching,*
*or a dog chasing its own tail.*
*It accompanies you every instant.*
*Don't believe in the reality*
*of good and bad experiences.*
*Although peace and happiness do not exist*
*as an actual thing or place, it is always available,*
*and they are like today's ephemeral weather,*
*like rainbows in the sky.*
*Wanting to grasp the ungraspable,*
*you exhaust yourself in vain.*
*As soon as you open and relax this tight fist of grasping,*
*infinite space is there – open, inviting and comfortable.*

*Make use of this spaciousness, this freedom and natural ease.*
*Don't search any further.*
*Don't go into the tangled jungle*
*looking for the great awakened elephant,*
*who is already resting quietly at home*
*in front of your own hearth.*
*Nothing to do or undo,*
*nothing to force,*
*nothing to want,*
*and nothing missing.*

*- Venerable Lama Gendun Rinpoche*

# CONTACT INFO

Raven Jones lives in Sonoma County, Northern California.

For Ayurvedic Consultations and Personal Cancer Coaching

with 'The Natural Cancer Recovery Program'

Email ravenayurveda@gmail.com

To purchase copies of this book or an online Ebook go to

www.myayurvedalife.com

CPSIA information can be obtained at www.ICGtesting.com
Printed in the USA
LVOW101553080113

314891LV00017B/753/P